Pineal Region Tumors

Guest Editors

ANDREW T. PARSA, MD, PhD
JEFFREY N. BRUCE, MD

NEUROSURGERY
CLINICS OF NORTH AMERICA

www.neurosurgery.theclinics.com

Consulting Editors
ANDREW T. PARSA, MD, PhD
PAUL C. McCORMICK, MD, MPH

July 2011 • Volume 22 • Number 3

SAUNDERS an imprint of ELSEVIER, Inc.

W.B. SAUNDERS COMPANY
A Division of Elsevier Inc.

1600 John F. Kennedy Blvd. • Suite 1800 • Philadelphia, PA 19103-2899

http://www.theclinics.com

NEUROSURGERY CLINICS OF NORTH AMERICA Volume 22, Number 3
July 2011 ISSN 1042-3680, ISBN-13: 978-1-4557-1112-3

Editor: Jessica McCool

Neurosurgery Clinics of North America (ISSN 1042-3680) is published quarterly by Elsevier Inc., 360 Park Avenue South, New York, NY 10010-1710. Months of issue are January, April, July, and October. Business and Editorial Offices: 1600 John F. Kennedy Blvd., Suite 1800, Philadelphia, PA 19103-2899. Customer Service Office: 11830 Westline Industrial Drive, St. Louis, MO 63146. Periodicals postage paid at New York, NY, and additional mailing offices. Subscription prices are $317.00 per year (US individuals), $492.00 per year (US institutions), $347.00 per year (Canadian individuals), $601.00 per year (Canadian institutions), $443.00 per year (international individuals), $601.00 per year (international institutions), $156.00 per year (US students), and $214.00 per year (international students). International air speed delivery is included in all *Clinics* subscription prices. All prices are subject to change without notice. **POSTMASTER:** Send address changes to *Neurosurgery Clinics of North America*, Elsevier Periodicals Customer Service, 11830 Westline Industrial Drive, St. Louis, MO 63146. **Customer Service: 1-800-654-2452 (US and Canada). From outside the US and Canada, call: 1-314-453-7041. Fax: 1-314-453-5170. E-mail: JournalsCustomerService-usa@elsevier.com (for print support) and journalsonlinesupport-usa@elsevier.com (for online support).**

Reprints. For copies of 100 or more, of articles in this publication, please contact the Commercial Reprints Department, Elsevier Inc., 360 Park Avenue South, New York, NY 10010-1710. Tel. (212) 633-3812; Fax: (212) 462-1935; E-mail: reprints@elsevier.com.

Neurosurgery Clinics of North America is covered in *MEDLINE/PubMed (Index Medicus)*, *EMBASE/Excerpta Medica*, and *Current Contents/Clinical Medicine (CC/CM)*.

Printed and bound by CPI Group (UK) Ltd, Croydon, CR0 4YY

Cover image copyright © 2011, The Johns Hopkins University. All rights reserved. Courtesy of Ian Suk, Johns Hopkins University; with permission.

Transferred to Digital Print 2011

Contributors

CONSULTING EDITORS

ANDREW T. PARSA, MD, PhD
Associate Professor, Principal Investigator,
Brain Tumor Research Center, Reza and
Georgianna Khatib Endowed Chair in Skull
Base Tumor Surgery, Department of
Neurological Surgery, University of California,
San Francisco, San Francisco, California

PAUL C. MCCORMICK, MD, MPH, FACS
Herbert & Linda Gallen Professor of
Neurological Surgery, Department of
Neurological Surgery, Columbia University
Medical Center, New York, New York

GUEST EDITORS

ANDREW T. PARSA, MD, PhD
Associate Professor, Principal Investigator,
Brain Tumor Research Center, Reza and
Georgianna Khatib Endowed Chair in Skull
Base Tumor Surgery, Department of
Neurological Surgery, University of California,
San Francisco, San Francisco, California

JEFFREY N. BRUCE, MD
Edgar M. Housepian Professor of Neurological
Surgery, Department of Neurological Surgery,
Columbia University College of Physicians and
Surgeons, New York, New York

AUTHORS

R.C.E. ANDERSON, MD
Department of Neurological Surgery,
Neurological Institute, Columbia University
Medical Center, New York, New York

DERICK ARANDA, MD
Department of Neurological Surgery, University
of California, San Francisco, San Francisco,
California

JEFFREY N. BRUCE, MD
Edgar M. Housepian Professor of Neurological
Surgery, Department of Neurological Surgery,
Columbia University College of Physicians and
Surgeons, New York, New York

OSAMAH CHOUDHRY, BA
Department of Neurological Surgery,
Neurological Institute of New Jersey,
New Jersey Medical School, University
of Medicine and Dentistry of New Jersey,
Newark, New Jersey

WINWARD CHOY, BA
Medical Student, Department of Neurological
Surgery, University of California, Los Angeles,
Los Angeles, California

AARON J. CLARK, MD, PhD
Department of Neurological Surgery, University
of California, San Francisco, San Francisco,
California

N. FELDSTEIN, MD
Department of Neurological Surgery,
Neurological Institute, Columbia University
Medical Center, New York, New York

E.J. FONTANA, MD
Department of Neurological
Surgery, Neurological Institute,
Columbia University Medical Center,
New York, New York

J. GARVIN, MD
Department of Oncology, Morgan Stanley
Children's Hospital of New York, Columbia
University Medical Center, New York,
New York

GAURAV GUPTA, MD
Department of Neurological Surgery,
Neurological Institute of New Jersey,
New Jersey Medical School, University
of Medicine and Dentistry of New Jersey,
Newark, New Jersey

SEUNGGU J. HAN, MD
Department of Neurological Surgery, University
of California, San Francisco, San Francisco,
California

SIMON J. HANFT, MD
Columbia University, New York, New York

STEVEN R. ISAACSON, MD
Columbia University, New York, New York

MICHAEL E. IVAN, MD
Department of Neurological Surgery, University
of California, San Francisco, San Francisco,
California

CHRISTOPHER JACKSON, BA
Departments of Neurosurgery and Oncology,
The Johns Hopkins University School of
Medicine, Baltimore, Maryland

GEORGE JALLO, MD
Associate Professor of Neurosurgery,
Pediatrics and Oncology, Departments of
Neurosurgery and Oncology, The Johns
Hopkins University School of Medicine,
Baltimore, Maryland

BENJAMIN C. KENNEDY, MD
Resident, Neurological Surgery, Columbia
University, New York, New York

WON KIM, MD
Neurosurgery Resident, Department of
Neurological Surgery, University of California,
Los Angeles, Los Angeles, California

MICHAEL LIM, MD
Assistant Professor of Neurosurgery and
Oncology, Departments of Neurosurgery and
Oncology, The Johns Hopkins University
School of Medicine, Baltimore, Maryland

JONATHON J. PARKER, BS
Department of Neurosurgery, University of
Colorado School of Medicine, Aurora, Colorado

ANDREW T. PARSA, MD, PhD
Associate Professor, Principal Investigator,
Brain Tumor Research Center, Reza and
Georgianna Khatib Endowed Chair in Skull
Base Tumor Surgery, Department of
Neurological Surgery, University of California,
San Francisco, San Francisco, California

ARIE PERRY, MD
Departments of Neurological Surgery and
Pathology, University of California,
San Francisco, San Francisco, California

**CHARLES J. PRESTIGIACOMO, MD,
FAANS, FACS**
Professor, Departments of Neurological
Surgery, Department of Radiology,
and Neurology and Neurosciences,
Neurological Institute of New Jersey,
New Jersey Medical School, University
of Medicine and Dentistry of New Jersey,
Newark, New Jersey

MARTIN J. RUTKOWSKI, BA
Department of Neurological Surgery, University
of California, San Francisco, San Francisco,
California

MARKO SPASIC, BA
Medical Student, Department of Neurological
Surgery, University of California, Los Angeles,
Los Angeles, California

MICHAEL E. SUGHRUE, MD
Director, Comprehensive Brain Tumor Center,
Department of Neurological Surgery, University
of Oklahoma, Oklahoma City, Oklahoma

MATTHEW C. TATE, MD, PhD
Department of Neurological Surgery, University
of California, San Francisco, San Francisco,
California

BRITTANY VOTH, BS
Research Assistant, Department of
Neurological Surgery, University of California,
Los Angeles, Los Angeles, California

ALLEN WAZIRI, MD
Assistant Professor, Department of
Neurosurgery, University of Colorado School
of Medicine, Aurora, Colorado

ISAAC YANG, MD
Assistant Professor, Department of Neurological Surgery; UCLA Brain Tumor Program, UCLA Department of Neurosurgery, University of California, Los Angeles, Los Angeles, California

ANDREW YEW, MD
Neurosurgery Resident, Department of Neurological Surgery, University of California, Los Angeles, Los Angeles, California

BRAD E. ZACHARIA, MD
Resident, Department of Neurological Surgery, Columbia University, New York, New York

Contents

On the Surgery of the Seat of the Soul: The Pineal Gland and the History of Its Surgical Approaches   321

Osamah Choudhry, Gaurav Gupta, and Charles J. Prestigiacomo

> The pineal gland has been studied through philosophy and science for thousands of years. Its role in human physiology was not well understood until the scientific community first started to report on pineal pathology in the eighteenth century. Throughout the nineteenth and twentieth centuries, reports on pineal tumors and the emergence of comparative anatomy allowed more complete understanding of pineal function. Neurosurgical methods of treating pineal pathology first emerged in the early twentieth century. In the latter half of the twentieth century, the emergence of microsurgical technique allowed for excellent outcomes with minimal morbidity and mortality.

Pathology of Pineal Parenchymal Tumors   335

Seunggu J. Han, Aaron J. Clark, Michael E. Ivan, Andrew T. Parsa, and Arie Perry

> Tumors of the pineal region can arise from multiple cellular origins and thus represent a very heterogeneous group of pathologies. Such tumors include pineal parenchymal tumors, germ cell tumors, astrocytomas, ependymomas, and papillary pineal tumors. Within the subgroup of pineal parenchymal tumors, there is a histopathologic spectrum ranging from pineocytoma to pineal parenchymal tumors of intermediate differentiation to pineoblastoma. The current World Health Organization classification and the pathologic features of each of the pineal parenchymal tumor subtypes are reviewed in this article.

Pineal Cyst: A Review of Clinical and Radiological Features   341

Winward Choy, Won Kim, Marko Spasic, Brittany Voth, Andrew Yew, and Isaac Yang

> Pineal cysts (PCs) are benign and often asymptomatic lesions of the pineal region that are typically small and do not change in size over time. PCs appear as small, well circumscribed, unilocular masses that either reside within or completely replace the pineal gland. This article reviews and discusses the characteristic features of PCs—clinical, histological, and identifiable by various imaging modalities—which assist clinicians in narrowing the differential diagnosis for pineal lesions.

Preoperative Evaluation of Pineal Tumors   353

Jonathon J. Parker and Allen Waziri

> The role of the neurosurgeon is critical for initiating preoperative evaluation and care for pineal region tumors. Preoperative evaluation of pineal region tumor can be simplified into a checklist: (1) evaluation for emergent surgical intervention due to symptomatic obstructive hydrocephalus or mass effect; (2) development of a focused differential after acquisition of craniospinal MRI, serum and cerebrospinal fluid oncoprotein levels, and cerebrospinal fluid cytology; and (3) decision on whether a biopsy,

surgical resection, or both are necessary. Subsequent biopsy or surgical resection is the first step of tumor management and leads to coordination of consultation with medical and radiation oncology.

Pineal region tumors represent 0.4% to 1.0% of intracranial tumors in American literature. Obtaining a tissue diagnosis is the cornerstone of the rational management of pineal lesions. The initial surgical decision involves choosing between a stereotactic biopsy and open microsurgical procedures. Open resection facilitates the maximal removal of tumor volume and has diagnostic accuracy and improved prognosis. Stereotactic biopsy is less invasive and has a lower risk of complications. A review of all major series reporting stereotactic biopsy for pineal region lesions reveals a mean diagnostic yield of 94%, with a morbidity of 1.3% and a mortality of 8.1%.

The pineal region can harbor highly diverse histologic tumor subtypes. Because optimal therapeutic strategies vary with tumor type, an accurate diagnosis is the foundation of enlightened management decisions. Either stereotactic biopsy or open surgery is essential for securing tissue for pathologic examination. Biopsy has the advantage of ease and minimal invasiveness but is associated with more sampling errors than open surgery. The emergence of endoscopic techniques and stereotactic radiosurgery provide complementary options to improve pineal tumor management, and will assume greater importance in the neurosurgeon's armamentarium.

The present review assesses how to make pineal surgery, refined over decades, better, ie, less invasive, while still respecting this delicate region, and achieving anatomic and oncologic goals. An explication of anatomic principles of this region, and some basic surgical principles of keyhole surgery are provided to further assist those interested in minimizing surgical impact during pineal surgery. Although this review, for the sake of brevity, focuses on the infratentorial-supracerebellar approach, many of these principles can be adapted to other approaches, such as the occipital transtentorial, without excessive imagination.

Intracranial GCTs are a heterogeneous group of neoplasms most commonly diagnosed in the pediatric population. Germinomas are exquisitely radiosensitive with long-term survival rates in excess of 90% with radiotherapy alone. NGGCTs are associated with a poorer prognosis and are typically treated with a combination of radiation and chemotherapy. Given the young age of these patients, achieving optimal outcomes will ultimately require a careful balance of maximizing disease control while minimizing adverse treatment effects. Here we review the management of intracranial GCTs and discuss the clinical outcomes of patients who undergo treatment for these rare and fascinating tumors.

Neurosurgery Clinics of North America

VISIT THE CLINICS ONLINE!

Access your subscription at:
www.theclinics.com

Preface

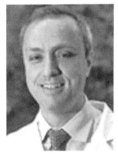 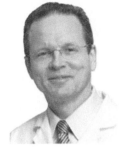

Andrew T. Parsa, MD, PhD   Jeffrey N. Bruce, MD
Guest Editors

Tumors of the pineal region are a challenging clinical entity that comprises a wide range of pathology. The advent of modern neurosurgical techniques, advanced preoperative imaging, endoscopy, and neuronavigation have dramatically improved the outcomes of surgically treated patients. In this issue of *Neurosurgery Clinics of North America*, the authors provide us with an excellent foundation for health care providers to build on. Historical elements relevant to the evolving management of pineal region tumor patients are discussed, followed by excellent reviews addressing the pathology, preoperative workup, radiosurgical, and surgical approaches to treatment. Outcomes for some of the most common pineal region tumors are elaborated on as well. Collectively we hope this issue serves as a guide for providers to develop a better understanding of these complex tumors.

Andrew T. Parsa, MD, PhD
Department of Neurological Surgery
University of California, San Francisco
505 Parnassus Avenue, M779, Box 0112
San Francisco, CA 94117, USA

Jeffrey N. Bruce, MD
Department of Neurological Surgery
Columbia University College of
Physicians and Surgeons
Room 434, Neurological Institute
Columbia University Medical Center
710 West 168th Street
New York, NY 10032, USA

E-mail addresses:
parsaa@neurosurg.ucsf.edu (A.T. Parsa)
jnb2@columbia.edu (J.N. Bruce)

doi:10.1016/j.nec.2011.06.002
1042-3680/11/$ – see front matter

neurosurgery.theclinics.com

On the Surgery of the Seat of the Soul: The Pineal Gland and the History of Its Surgical Approaches

Osamah Choudhry, BA[a,1], Gaurav Gupta, MD[a,1], Charles J. Prestigiacomo, MD, FAANS[a,b,c,*]

KEYWORDS

- Pineal gland • Pineal tumors • History of neurosurgery
- Pineal surgery

Strategically located at one of the most difficult central nervous system access points, it is not surprising to see why the pineal gland has enjoyed a somewhat mysterious and mystical history. Unlike other vertebrates, humans are not as directly dependent on photoperiodicity as a mechanism of survival advantage. Aberrations in circadian rhythm, however, as evidenced by several diseases, such as seasonal affective disorder and Smith-Magenis syndrome, can affect lives and livelihoods. The growth in understanding of the pineal gland, its function, its relevance, and the ability to treat its diseases has been slowed by many natural and derived challenges. These challenges provide the backdrop against which this gland's interesting history is shaped.

EARLY DESCRIPTIONS OF THE PINEAL GLAND

The pineal gland has been the subject of human inquiry for thousands of years. The name itself is derived from the Latin word, *pinealis*, with *pinea* meaning pinecone, a reference to the shape of the gland because it hangs from the posterior roof of the third ventricle. It has also been referred to as the *epiphysis* ("that which grows on something") as well as the *konareion* (meaning in Greek, "the cone of the pine tree").[1] In much of the Latin literature, it has been referred to as turbo, corpus turbinatus, glandula turbinate, glandula piniformis, glandula conoides, conariumm, penis cerebri, corpus pineale, and virga cerebri. In the German literature, it is referred to as Zirbel and Zirbeldrüse.[2]

Interest in the pineal gland can be traced as far back as ancient China during the reign of the Yellow Emperor (2697–2597 BC).[3] In the ancient Hindu scriptures, the *Vedas*, a collection of religious teachings of ancient India, the pineal gland was 1 of the 7 chakra points, or centers of vital energy. Specifically, the pineal gland was considered the "supreme or crown chakra...the ultimate center of spiritual force."[4,5]

The Greek physician and philosopher, Aelius Galenus (130–200 AD), better known as Galen of Pergamon (**Fig. 1**), credits Herophilus (325–280 BC)

Conflicts and disclosures: The authors have nothing to disclose.

[a] Department of Neurological Surgery, Neurological Institute of New Jersey, New Jersey Medical School, University of Medicine and Dentistry of New Jersey, 90 Bergen Street, Suite 8100, Newark, NJ 07101-1709, USA

[b] Department of Radiology, New Jersey Medical School, University of Medicine and Dentistry of New Jersey, 90 Bergen Street, Suite 8100, Newark, NJ 07101-1709, USA

[c] Department of Neurology and Neurosciences, Neurological Institute of New Jersey, New Jersey Medical School, University of Medicine and Dentistry of New Jersey, 90 Bergen Street, Suite 8100, Newark, NJ 07101-1709, USA

[1] Authors contributed equally to this work.

* Corresponding author.

E-mail address: presticj@umdnj.edu

Neurosurg Clin N Am 22 (2011) 321–333

doi:10.1016/j.nec.2011.04.001

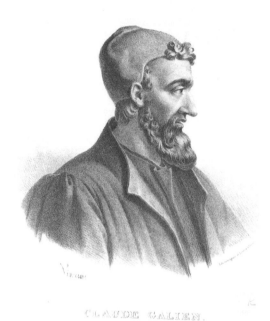

Fig. 1. Galen; lithograph by Pierre Roche Vigneron (Paris: Lith de Gregoire et Deneux, approximately 1865). (*Courtesy of* History of Medicine Division, National Library of Medicine.)

as the first to discover the pineal gland.[6] Herophilus, a Greek physician at the University of Alexandria in Egypt, is considered the first person to have systematically performed scientific dissections of cadavers, recording his findings in 9 volumes. Herophilus asserted that the pineal gland was a valve or sphincter controlling the flow of pneuma from the third to the fourth ventricles. Pneuma was considered the fine substance derived from air and responsible for thought (*psycikon*, in Greek) and organic movement.[7,8]

Galen himself did not entertain such respect for the pineal gland, considering it merely a supporting structure for the deep venous structures/internal cerebral veins. In his writings, he scoffs at Herophilus' ideas on the pineal gland[9]:

> The notion that the pineal body is what regulates the passage of the pneuma is the opinion of those who are ignorant of the action of the vermiform epiphysis [vermis superior cerebelli] and who give more than due credit to this gland.

Galen found Herophilus' hypothesis of the pineal gland's function as a valve to control flow of pneuma laughable. In the eighth book of his anatomic works, *De Usu Partim (On The Usefulness of the Parts of the Body)*,[10] he asserts that the external nature of the gland with respect to the interventricular space meant it could have no

such role. Galen advocated that it was the vermis of the cerebellum that regulated the passage of pneuma from the third to the fourth ventricle. Galen's view went unchallenged throughout the Medieval Period. Not until the fifteenth century was the pineal gland re-examined. During the Renaissance, Andreas Vesalius (1514–1564), the father of modern anatomy, topographically mapped the pineal gland and discussed the relevant anatomy in *De Humani Corporis Fabrica, Libri Septem (On the Fabric of the Human Body)*,[11,12] first published in 1543. In regards to possible pineal function, he agreed with Galen's viewpoint of the insignificance of the gland due to its exterior location. During the same time, Niccolò Massa (1485–1569), an Italian anatomist, in 1536 proved that the ventricles were not filled with pneuma but with liquor cerebro-spinalis, or the cerebrospinal fluid.[13]

The Pineal Gland—The Seat of the Soul?

In the seventeenth century the French logician and philosopher, René Descartes (1596–1650) (**Fig. 2**), a contemporary of Vesalius, studied and wrote extensively on the pineal gland. Descartes, although widely known for his work in mathematics and philosophy, was no stranger to human anatomy. To the pineal gland he gave the unique distinction of "the seat of man's soul." The first description of the pineal in his works is documented

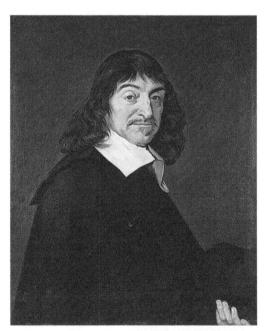

Fig. 2. René Descartes; oil painting by Frans Hals, 1649; in the Louvre, Paris. (*Courtesy of* Cliché Musées Nationaux, Paris.)

in *Dioptrics* (1637) as a small gland (or the *conarion*) in the middle of the ventricles, the seat of the *sensus communis* (the general faculty of the senses).[14] He maintained the pineal gland was the organ that allowed the *res cogitans* (spirit or anima) to maintain contact with the *res extensa* (the material body*).* In his *Les Passions de l'Âme (The Passions of the Soul),*[15] from 1649, he writes, "Although the soul is joined with the entire body, there is one part of the body [the pineal] in which it exercises its function more than elsewhere…"

In Descartes' philosophy, the pineal body was the medium between the soul and the body. Descartes argued that the pineal gland served as a filter that accumulated *espirits animaux* (animal spirits) from the blood. This spirit was then distributed through tiny pores in the ventricular walls to nerves attached to motor nerves based on the movement of the pineal gland. Information received from the eyes and optic nerves was passed along to the pineal gland along the ventricular pores and used as input corresponding to resultant pineal gland motor output (**Fig. 3**). In *L' Homme (Treatise of Man),*[16] he explains his reasoning for why the pineal is the seat of the soul. He believed it was the only structure in the

entire brain that was not duplicated. He notes that the pineal is small, light, and easily movable and even though the other gland (ie, the pituitary) is also small and undivided, it is immobile and located outside the brain. Using the same analogy, he said that Galen's vermian appendage was not a suitable candidate because it had 2 halves.

Other scientists of the Renaissance also held unique views on pineal function. François Magendie (1783–1855), a French physiologist, advocated that the pineal gland itself acts like a tampon, designed to expand or shrink and in this way close off or open the aqueduct of Sylvius. Gunz (1753) attributed dementia to impeding flow of the spirits caused by the pineal body.[2]

By the early to mid-nineteenth century, the relatively new field of comparative anatomy was emerging. Scientists compared structures in the human body with those found in various classes of the animal kingdom, including vertebrates and nonvertebrates. Ahlborn[17] and Rabl-Rückhardt (1839–1906),[6,18] both accomplished comparative anatomists, pointed out the similarity between the nonmammalian pineal gland and the primary optic vesicles. Other scientists, including De Graaf[19,20] and Korschelt and Spencer,[21] described the

A

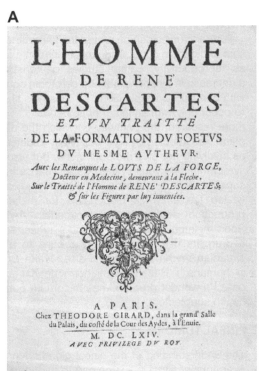

B

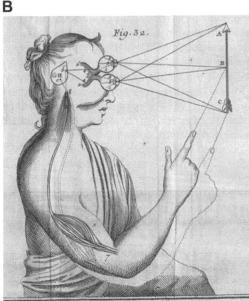

Fig. 3. (*A*) René Descartes' *L'Homme (Treatise of Man)*. Published in 1664, posthumously, by Descartes' self-appointed literary executor, Claude Clerselier. (*B*) A drawing from René Descartes' *L'Homme*, showing the pineal gland (H) as the link between visual stimuli and resulting action. (*Courtesy of* Historical Collections & Services, Claude Moore Health Sciences Library, University of Virginia.)

reptilian and amphibian epiphysis as a unique photosensory organ, whose function regressed and became vestigial in mammals.

Its role as a third eye in nonmammals sparked an immense scientific output on its possible role in humans but also led to an important role in religious thought. An example of this is from Helena Blavatsky (1831–1891), the founder of theosophy. She advocated the ancient Hindu concept of the third eye of Shiva, the ambaka, through which communication in humans is done. For Madame Blavatsky, humans received this divine inspiration not through a figurative third eye but literally through the pineal gland itself. It was an "organ of spiritual vision."[22]

Greater understanding of the pineal was made with the advancement in the field of microscopic histology. Kölliker in 1888 demonstrated that the pineal gland was mainly composed of 2 type of cells—the small round cells and the multipolar nerve cells with the compact bundle of nerve cells.[23] Perhaps the greatest leap forward in understanding the pineal gland came from Studnicka in first decade of the twentieth century. He pushed forward the hypothesis that the pineal body had glandular function based on the activity of its nonmammalian well-developed counterpart.[5] Within the mammalian pineal gland, he distinguished the pinealocyte from the neuroglial cells, suggesting that the vesicles and granules present within the pinealocyte hinted at their secretory activity.[21] Studnicka's claims were taken with all the more seriousness once the first case reports emerged at the end of the nineteenth century, suggesting a relation between a boy with a pinealoma and precocious puberty.[24] Cajal thought that the nerve fibers in the pineal body are sympathetic and the body itself a vascular gland.[23] Marburg, during the first decade of the twentieth century, advanced the principle of the pineal gland regulating hormonal cycles. Having coined the term, *pubertas praecox* (precocious puberty), he explained that this occurred due to hypopinealism or destruction of pineal glandular tissue by a tumor, such as a pinealoma. Likewise, Marburg hypothesized that hyperpinealism resulted in slow and incomplete development of the reproductive organs.[25–28] Other researchers even touted the use of pineal gland extract for antigonadotropic purposes.[6,29,30]

This view, however, was largely discounted in the 1930s and 1940s, as researchers understood more about the structure and function of the hypothalamus. It was observed that pinealomas affected sexual development not intrinsically but through mechanical force on specific hypothalamic centers.[31] In the 1940s further research continued with Bargmann's landmark article

describing the anatomy and histology of the pineal gland as well as commenting on external and internal factors, which could induce changes in pineal function. Specifically, and importantly, he mentioned the need for further research for the influence of light on pineal secretions. Bargmann also suggested the pineal to not only have hormonal input and output but also neural input and output.[6,32]

During World War II (1940s), with the advent of the electron microscope, the mammalian pineal gland was confirmed as having neurosecretory cells, named pinealocytes, and supporting glial cells. The visualization of the endoplasmic reticulum and dense core vesicles also revealed more about the pineal's secretory functions.[33,34]

The Discovery and Purification of Melatonin

In 1958, Aaron B. Lerner (1921–2007), chair of the Yale University Department of Dermatology, isolated a potential pineal hormone known for its curious effect of lightening skin when fed to amphibians. The compound, N-acetyl-5-methoxy-tryptamine, was shown to have a blanching effect on dermal melanophores. He named it, *melatonin*, from the Greek *melas* (black) and *tonoes* (to labor).[35–37] Soon after the discovery of melatonin, the biosynthesis via tryptophan and the enzymes involved in the process were isolated.[38,39]

Further studies demonstrated the importance of light and dark in controlling pineal function as well as reproductivity. Earlier studies demonstrated a decrease in pineal weight and serotonin content with continuous illumination.[40,41] This was shown to occur only with an intact optic nerve.[42–44] With more research, the pathway by which the pineal gland was affected by light was finally understood as involving not only the optic nerve but also the sympathetic nervous system via a synapse in the superior cervical ganglion.[45,46] Other studies revealed the enzymes responsible for melatonin production demonstrated a circadian rhythm. Soon melatonin was isolated and synthesized as a drug. Its use demonstrated abilities to affect circadian rhythm and normal sleep/wake cycles in humans.[47] Recently, the hormone has been called a wonder drug and has become a popular health supplement.

PINEAL TUMORS

The understanding of the pineal gland's function over time was tied in a large part to the pathology encountered and reported in the literature.

Charles Drelincourt (1633–1697), a French physician, was the first to report a case of pineal tumor in the seventeenth century. As reported by

Magnet in a book published in Geneva in 1717, Drelincourt encountered a 20-year-old woman with a hardened pineal gland found the size of "a fowl's egg."[37,48]

Giovanni Battista Morgagni (1682–1771), an Italian anatomist and the father of modern anatomic pathology, also recorded cases of various patients with enlarged pineal glands. In his famous compendium of pathology, *The Seats and Causes of Disease*, published in 1761, he went into a discussion on the calcified pineal gland and reported on a patient with a calcified gland the size of an egg.[49]

Gilbert Blane (1749–1834), a Scottish physician, was the first in the English-speaking to report a pineal tumor. He served as physician of the British fleet for more than 35 years and was known for his efforts in instituting the mandatory use of lemon juice to prevent scurvy. He reported on a pineal tumor in a 36-year-old naval officer.[37,50] The tumor was found to press down on the cerebellum, resulting in excruciating pain and eventual delirium.[51]

Throughout the nineteenth century, other case reports emerged on tumors of the pineal region but little could be reported in regards to histology because microscopic tissue examination had yet to be perfected.[52] Only gross pathology could be described, resulting in various inaccurate names given to pineal tumors, including adenomas, carcinomas, sarcoma, and gliomas.

In 1883, the French ophthalmologist, Henri Parinaud (1844–1905), described a syndrome characterized by supranuclear paralysis of vertical gaze seen in 10 of his patients.[53] He was unable, however, to accurately pinpoint the anatomic location responsible for the syndrome. Parinaud syndrome is thought to be caused by the compression of the mesencephalic tectum by an enlarging pineal mass.

The first pineal tumor correctly identified and studied was the teratoma. Karl Weigert (1845–1904), a German pathologist from Breslau, is credited with correctly identifying its gross and microscopic histology. In 1875, Weigert reported on a 14-year-old boy with a pineal teratoma, which histologically consisted of squamous and columnar epithelium along with hair and skin.[54]

In 1896, Richard Gutzeit first commented on a possible relationship between the pineal teratoma and endocrine abnormalities. In his dissertation for his Doctor of Medicine degree, he described a 7-year-old boy with unusually large and developmentally mature external genitalia and a concurrent pineal teratoma.[55] In 1899, 2 further articles reported on the peculiar association between precocious puberty and pineal teratomas. The second article was

presented at a Pathologic Society of London meeting.[37,56,57]

By 1909, the relationship between precocious puberty and pineal tumors, in particular the teratoma, was established. Two articles were crucial in this regard. Lothar von Frankl-Hochwart (1872–1914),[58] a distinguished neurologist from Vienna, presented a case report of a pineal teratoma and thoroughly discussed its relation with precocious puberty. In 1910, Giovanni Pellizzi of Pisa, Italy, reported on precocious genital development with a pineal tumor, which came to be referred to as Pellizzi syndrome, in a 2-part article in an Italian journal.[59] Not only was precocious puberty described in relation to pineal teratomas but also hypogonadism discussed. The first case report discussing this was by Max Neumann of Karlsruhe in 1901.[60]

In the late nineteenth and early twentieth centuries, terms for pineal tumors had been borrowed from histologic variants of tumors they resembled in other parts of the body. Knud H. Krabbe (1885–1965),[61] a Danish neurologist from Copenhagen, in his landmark thesis, *Histologic Studies of the Pineal Body*, published in 1912, was the first to use the word the word, *pinealoma*. His extensive study and dissection of more than 400 human postmortem pineal glands led him to conclude that the normal gland was composed of essentially 2 cell lines—special pineal cells and neuroglial cells. In general, the term pinealoma was intended to be used for a generic pineal mass. The technical limitations of the era led many scientists to falsely conclude the tumors were all of pineal parenchymal origin.[37]

Gilbert Horrax (1887–1957), an American neurosurgeon, and Percival Bailey (1892–1973), an American neuropathologist, neurosurgeon, and psychiatrist, in 1925 subdivided pineal tumors into 2 groups.[62] Their first group had 11 cases of a tumor cell type that resembled the adult pineal parenchymal cells. This group was entitled, pinealomas, as Krabbe had proposed. The second group consisted of 2 cases of teratomas. The following year Bailey and Harvey Cushing (1869–1939) subdivided the first group into pineoblastomas and pinealomas.[63] They observed that the pinealoblastoma resembled a cerebellar medulloblastoma, a tumor they first described 2 years previously in 1924.[64] Pinealoblastomas were described as rapidly growing tumors of the pineal body consisting of primitive glial cells or spongioblasts. Pinealomas, in contrast, were described as made of large spherical cells with processes ending in bulbs. The newly named pinealoblastoma was quickly accepted by other pathologists, including Russell and Rubinstein[65] and Ziilch.[66]

The second tumor, pinealoma, however, had controversy surrounding its exact classification and histopathologic structure. Bailey had originally described the tumor as composed of neoplastic pineal parenchymal cells and lymphoid cells in a fibrovascular stroma.[63]

Joseph Globus[67] (1885–1952) of Mount Sinai Hospital, New York, agreed with Bailey but asserted the lymphoid cells were also neoplastic. He considered the tumor an "autochthonous teratoid of bidermal origin." In a differing point of view, Dorothy H. Russell of London Hospital felt the tumors were *atypical teratomas*—a term once used to describe testicular teratomas.[37,68] Nathan B. Friedman[69] of the US Armed Forces Institute of Pathology in Washington, DC, agreed with Russell. He was convinced that histopathologically the tumor was similar if not identical to the seminoma of the testes, dysgerminoma of the ovaries, and extragonadal germinomas. For this group of similar tumors, whether they were genital or extragenital in location, he coined the term, *germinoma*. Thus, for more than 30 years the term pinealoma was used for the most common pineal tumor, today known as the germinoma.

Eventually, by the 1970s, it had been documented that all varieties of germ cell tumors had the potential to be found in the pineal region. Although germinomas and teratomas are the most prevalent, choriocarcinoma, yolk sac tumor, and embryonal carcinoma have all been found.[37,70,71]

The term, pinealoma, was found to cause confusion and after Friedman introduced the term, germinoma, pinealoma fell out of favor. A new term was needed to describe well-differentiated pineal parenchymal tumors. In 1933, the term, *pineocytoma*, was conferred on a "better differentiated pinealocytic tumor" by Pio del Rio-Hortega (1882–1945) of Buenos Aires.[37,72] By 1959, Russell and Rubinstein adopted pineocytoma for a "differentiated pineal parenchymal neoplasm" in their textbook.[65] They also explicitly demonstrated the relationship between rosette formations and pineocytomas. Later, other investigators went further and differentiated pineocytomas into 2 categories, including a pure, monomorphic variant composed of confluent pineocytomatous rosettes and the more common mixed pineocytomas with pineocytomatous rosettes and "neoplastic ganglion and glial cells."[37]

Russell and Rubinstein's textbook, *Pathology of Tumors of the Nervous System*, became the standard for the classification of pineal tumors. They divided pineal masses into 4 broad categories: tumors of germ cell origin (germinomas and teratomas), tumors of pineal parenchymal cells (pineoblastomas and pineocytomas), tumors of glial and other cell origin, and non-neoplastic cysts and masses.[65]

HISTORICAL ASPECTS OF PINEAL TUMOR SURGERY

> *Pineal tumors are perhaps the most dangerous of all intracranial tumors to attack surgically.*
>
>   —*Walter E. Dandy*[73]

The pineal gland's deep intracranial location and close relationship to the deep venous system of the brain made surgery difficult and often resulted in a high rate of morbidity and mortality. Eventually the tumors were considered unresectable and progress was made only by treatment with conventional radiotherapy.[74]

The first known attempt at pineal tumor resection was undertaken by the pioneering British surgeon Sir Victor Horsley (1857–1916) in 1910.[75,76] Horsely, Victor described an infratentorial approach to the pineal gland. He never claimed success and the patient passed away from surgical complications. Conrad M.H. Howell (1877–1960), who presented in 1910 at the Royal Society of Medicine on *Tumors of the Pineal Body*, described Horsely's comments on his surgical efforts[75]:

With regard…to the possibility of doing anything surgically, he was bound to confess that the surgical results so far were far from favorable. He thought that this might be due to the fact that he had approached the lesion subtentorially. In the next case with which he has to deal he would certainly go supratentorially splitting the tentorium from the centro-posterior position and exposing the tumor in that manner…

Brunner made his attempt in 1913 at pineal tumor surgery occurred soon after.[77,78] His patient was a 27-year-old man in an asylum for history of hebephrenia (disorganized schizophrenia) who suddenly developed characteristic signs of an intracranial mass lesion, including cerebellar ataxia and eye movement disturbances. Brunner opened a skin flap over the posterior fossa but the patient unfortunately died during the second stage of the operation. One year later, the patient's 27-year-old cousin coincidentally presented with the same signs and symptoms of an intracranial mass of the quadrigeminal region.[77,78] The surgeon chose a completely different approach, this time through the posterior corpus callosum. The approach provided a limited view of the tumor and severe venous hemorrhage forced Brunner to abandon the operation before all of the tumor could be removed. The patient did recover but had significant sensory symptoms, presumably due to the callosotomy.

In 1913, the first successful operation in the pineal region was reported by Hermann Oppenheim (1858–1919), who had referred a patient to Fedor Krause (1857–1937), a German surgeon.[79] The patient was a 10-year-old boy with a neoplasm diagnosed within the pineal region. The operation was performed in a sitting position. Krause used a broad flap to expose both sides of the cerebellum and used the infratentorial-supracerebellar approach (**Fig. 4**). He opened the dura, holding the upper part up with a spatula. The contents of the posterior fossa, including the cerebellar hemispheres, "prolapsed posteriorly into the operation field." The plane between the upper cerebellar vermis and lower tentorium was divided to expose the tumor. Using a medium-sharp curette, Krause was successfully able to remove the tumor completely. On removal, the left and right internal cerebral veins were visualized. The dura was sutured, allowing the prolapsed cerebellum to be kept within its original position. The tumor was described as a well-encapsulated sarcoma. The operation was a resounding success with the boy free of all complaints. The only abnormality on physical examination was dysdiadochokinesia in the left hand. The advantage of using this intrafentorial-supracerebellar approach was that a cerebellar tumor could be recognized if a misdiagnosis occurred. More importantly it allowed a surgeon to avoid the deep venous system situated dorsal and lateral to the pineal region to avoid injury to the deep veins, which was the main cause of surgical morbidity.[76,80]

Water E. Dandy published his experience with pineal region surgery in 1915.[81] He experimented

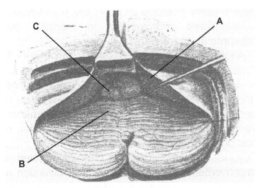

Fig. 4. Illustration of Krause's novel approach to the pineal region though an infratentorial (A) supratentorial (B) route revealing the pineal lesion (C). (*From* Oppenheim H, Krause F. Operative Erfolge bei Geschwülsten der Sehhügel—und Vierhügelgegend. Berl Klin Wochenschr 1913;50:2316–22; with permission.)

with several approaches to the pineal region in dogs (**Fig. 5**). His method included an anteroposterior exposure of the pineal, which was then removed with a small rongeur. It required opening the third ventricle due to the pineal body's close attachment to the ventricle's posterior wall. All 12 dogs he operated on could not survive the operation. All were found to have ventricles filled with blood.[76]

In 1921, Dandy published a case report of 3 patients using his parieto-occipital transcallosal approach. He used a large parieto-occipital bone flap and on separating and retracting the cerebral hemispheres a 3- to 4-cm incision in the exposed corpus callosum with further retraction brought the tumor into complete view (**Fig. 6**). Although there were no perioperative fatalities, none of the patients survived past 1 year.[76,82] Walker soon perfected the approach and by 1936 had published 10 more cases. By then, Walker's technique was accepted by the surgical community as the favored approach to the pineal region. His neurology partner at Johns Hopkins, however, reported a disorder of higher cortical function postoperatively when using this approach. Patients emerged with a disorder known as alexia without agraphia.[83]

In 1929, Max Peet removed a 1.5-cm fibrous pineal tumor via Dandy's parieto-occipital transcallosal approach. Radiation was used postoperatively. The patient was followed-up 31 years postoperatively and found doing well, working as a painter. This was considered at the time the second successful total gross resection of a pineal tumor (after Krause's work).[84,85]

The third successful complete removal of a pineal tumor is credited to Otfrid Foerster (1873–1941).[86] In 1928, he reported a technique involving an occipital craniotomy after which lateral ventricle puncture was used to allow for decompression and retraction of the occipital lobe from the falx and tentorium. The tumor was then brought into view and carefully resected. In the case of insufficient exposure, the falx and splenium could also be incised. He reported on 3 patients operated on with this technique. The first was a 25-year-old man who was operated on in 1927 with total removal of the glioma achieved. The second patient had initially been operated on in 1923 with a partial removal of the cystic tumor. The second operation found the recurrent mass densely adherent to the midbrain and again only a partial removal was possible. The patient died postoperatively 2 days later. In the third case, although signs of a pineal region tumor were present on exposure, no tumor and no pineal gland were visualized.

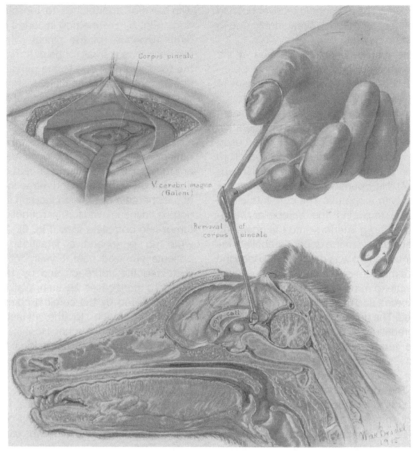

Fig. 5. Illustration of Dandy's experimental technique to extirpate the pineal body in dogs. (*From* Dandy WE. Extirpation of the pineal body. J Exp Med 1915;22:237–7; with permission.)

Nevertheless the patient recovered neurologically and endocrinologically.[76,86]

Van Wagenen, in 1931,[87] described a novel approach to pineal tumor surgery. He used a dilated right lateral ventricle to gain exposure to a "spongioblastic type" tumor in a 34-year-old woman (**Fig. 7**). The ventricle's thin medial wall was divided with electrocautery exposing the tumor. All of it was safely removed except for a small amount adherent to large adjoining veins. Postoperatively the patient's course was uneventful and "she remained entirely free from symptoms of hydrocephalus for 15 months following surgery."[76,87]

By 1950, the favored approach was conservative tumor treatment by decompression and radiation therapy rather than radical tumor extirpation. Mortality rates were high, ranging from 20% to 70% when using invasive surgery.[73,88,89] James L. Poppen (1903–1978), a pioneer in surgical approaches to the pineal area, and Marino favored "X-ray therapy unless unusually critical conditions necessitate immediate surgical intervention."[90] Ward and Spurling collected 14 cases of pineal tumors treated by subtemporal decompression and irradiation.[91] Six patients were alive and well past 5 years postoperation. At the time this was a significant improvement in mortality over attempts at direct surgical excision.

Another conservative method introduced by Arne Torkildsen (1899–1968) was the procedure of ventriculocisternostomy.[92] He first published on it in 1948 describing 8 cases in which he diverted the obstructed spinal fluid from the lateral ventricle to the cistern magna with a catheter. He had only 1 operative death and 3 patients survived beyond 2 years. This idea eventually led to improvements in cerebrospinal fluid diversion resulting in ventriculoatrial and ventriculoperitoneal shunts commonly used along with irradiation of the tumor region.[93]

In 1956, Bohuslav Zapletal revived Krause's infratentorial-supracerebellar approach with publication of his experience on 4 patients.[94] This

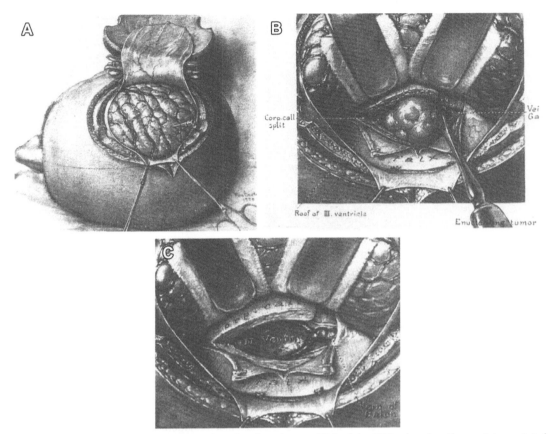

Fig. 6. Dandy's technique for accessing the pineal region, published in 1921, showing the parieto-occipital opening with retraction of the dural flap (*A*) and exposure of the tumor via division of the corpus callosum (*B*) and visualization of the third ventricle and deep cerebral veins after tumor removal (*C*). (*From* Dandy WE. An operation for the removal of pineal tumors. Surg Gynecol Obstet 1921;33:113–9. Reprinted with permission from the *Journal of the American College of Surgeons*, formerly *Surgery Gynecology & Obstetrics*.)

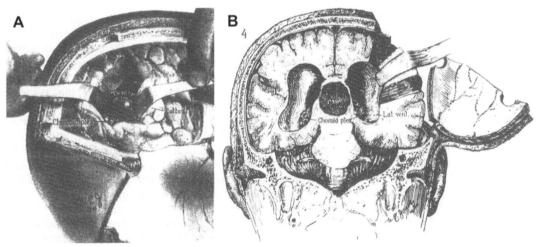

Fig. 7. (*A*, *B*) Van Wagenen's approach to the pineal region through a dilated lateral ventricle. (*From* Van Wagenen W. A surgical approach for the removal of certain pineal tumors. Surg Gyn Obst 1931;53:216–20. Reprinted with permission from the *Journal of the American College of Surgeons*, formerly *Surgery Gynecology & Obstetrics*.)

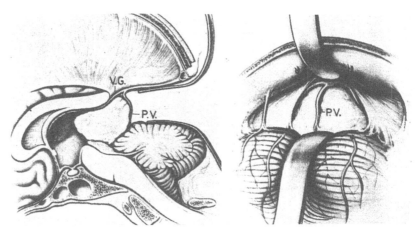

Fig. 8. Drawing of Stein's infratentorial supracereballar approach to pineal tumors. (*From* Stein BM. The infratentorial supracerebellar approach to pineal lesions. J Neurosurg 1971;35(2):197–2; with permission.)

method became more popular when Bennett M. Stein,[95] Chairman and Professor of Neurosurgery at Columbia University College of Physicians and Surgeons, reported 6 cases of operations with the same approach. Performed in the sitting position, a suboccipital craniectomy was performed extending to the transverse sinus, with the arch of C1 removed (**Fig. 8**). Using the operating microscope, the quadrigeminal region was exposed after cutting the arachnoid. Stein was able to perform the cases with no perioperative mortality and little morbidity.

By the 1960s, the 2 most common surgical approaches were the infratentorial-supracerebellar route and the occipital transtentorial or transcallosal approach.[96–102]

By the 1970s, the development of microneurosurgical techniques, use of the operating microscope, and the progression of neurologic critical care allowed for use of radical approaches to the pineal region to be performed with minimal morbidity and mortality. In addition, the introduction and development of stereotaxy improved access to the region for biopsies, allowing more specific treatment targeting certain tumor types.

More recently, the use of newer endoscopic techniques have led to a fresh approach to pineal tumor excision.[103–105] Endoscopy has replaced most other methods as the preferred approach to biopsy of pineal masses. Its use in the pineal region was first described by Fukishima and colleagues[106] in 1973. Concerns with venous hemorrhage and lack of techniques for hemostasis limited the use of the endoscope in the pineal region during the 1970s and early 1980s.[107,108] In 1997, Robinson and Cohen[109] first described endoscopic biopsy combined with endoscopic third ventriculocisternostomy as an alternative to

inserting a ventriculoperitoneal shunt and performing a separate biopsy using stereotactical or microsurgical technique. The advantage of this in the management of a pineal mass included direct visualization of the tumor, simultaneous treatment of hydrocephalus, and reduction procedural morbidity with a combination of diagnostic and therapeutic procedures.[107] Endoscopic biopsy with third ventriculostomy is commonly used in the initial management of a pineal mass.

Although pineal region surgery is not trivial, in the past 25 years rate of major morbidity and mortality have dropped to 0% to 2% in published surgical series.[74] Newer techniques for surgical management of pineal masses undoubtedly will be developed in the future.

SUMMARY

The pineal gland holds a unique place in human civilization. At various points throughout history, it has had lofty attributes ascribed to it by religious traditions and classical philosophy. Little was known about the pineal gland's actual functions until serious investigation into the pathology encountered with it occurred. From there, an evolution in science and technology allowed scientists to understand its basic attributes. As pineal tumors continued to be reported in the literature during the nineteenth and twentieth centuries, neurosurgery eventually started to play an important role in the management of pineal pathology. Among the earlier neurosurgeons, pineal tumors were feared and respected for being located in arguably one of the most dangerous and inaccessible areas within the cranial vault. Technology and the collective strength of will and character have emboldened neurosurgeons to successfully approach and treat lesions in that which was once considered the seat of the soul.

REFERENCES

1. Erlich SS, Apuzzo ML. The pineal gland: anatomy, physiology, and clinical significance. J Neurosurg 1985;63(3):321–41.
2. Tilney F, Warren LF. The morphology and evolutional significance of the pineal body; being part I of a contribution to the study of the epiphysis cerebri with an interpretation of the morphological, physiological and clinical evidence. Philadelphia: The Wistar Institute of Anatomy and Biology; 1919.
3. Veith I. The yellow emperor's classic of internal medicine. Berkeley and Los Angeles (CA): University of California Press; 2002.
4. Reiter R, Robinson J. Melatonin: your body's natural wonder drug. New York (NY): Bantam Books; 1995.
5. Kappers J. Structure and functions of the epiphysis cerebri progress in Brain Research, vol. 10. New York (NY): Elsevier; 1965.
6. Kappers JA. Short history of pineal discovery and research. In: Kappers JA, Pévet P, editors, Progress in brain research, vol. 52. New York (NY): Elsevier; 1979. p. 3–22.
7. Roux P. Contribution a vetude de la glande pineale ou epiphyse. Paris: Fac Sc Univ; 1937.
8. Mettler CC, Mettler FA. History of medicine: a correlative text, arranged according to subjects. Philadelphia (PA): Blakiston; 1947.
9. May MT. Galen on the usefulness of the parts of the body: peri chreias moriōn [romanized form] de usu partium. Ithaca (NY): Cornell University Press; 1968.
10. May MT. On the usefulness of parts of the body (de usu partium translator for original author— Galen). Ithaca (NY): Cornell University Press; 1968.
11. Vesalius A. De humani corporis fabrica libri septem. Basilae: Joannis Oporini; 1543.
12. Vesalius A, Richardson W, Carman J. On the fabric of the human body: book VI the heart and associated organs, book VII the brain. San Francisco (CA): Norman Publishers; 2009.
13. Massa N, Weber G. Liber introductorius anatomiae. Leo. S. Firenze (Italy): Olschki; 2006.
14. Descartes R. La dioptrique. Oeuvres de Descartes. V. Cousin. F. G. Levrault 5. Paris (France); 1824.
15. Descartes R, 1649, (In French). Les passions de l'âme. Amsterdam (Holland): Chez Louys & Daniel Elzevier; 1649.
16. Descartes R. L'homme. Treatise of man. In: Clerselier C, editor. Treatise of Man. Paris: Jacques le Gras; 1664. p. 199. [in French].
17. Ahlborn F. Uber die bedeutung der zirbeldriise (glandula pinealis, commissur, Epiphysis cerebri). Z Zool 1884;40:331–7.
18. Rabl-Rückhardt H. Ur deutung der zirbeldruse (epiphyse). Zool Anz 1886;9:536–47.
19. De Graaf HW. Bijdrage tot de kennis van den bouw en de ontwikkeling der epiphyse by amphibien en reptilien. Thesis. Leyden; 1886.
20. De Graaf HW. Zur anatomie und entwicklung der epiphyse bei amphibien und reptilien. Zool Anz 1886;9:191–4.
21. Studnicka FK, Oppel A, editors, Die parictalorgane. Lehrbuch der vergleichenden mikro- skopischen anatomie, vol. 5. Verlag Berlin (Germany): Springer; 1905.
22. Blavatsky HP. The secret doctrine: the synthesis of science, religion, and philosophy. London: Theosophical Publishing Co; 1888.
23. Tilney F, Warren LF. The morphology and evolutional significance of the pineal body; being part I of a contribution to the study of the epiphysis cerebri with an interpretation of the morphological, physiological and clinical evidence. Philadelphia (PA). The Wistar Institute of Anatomy and Biology 1919;1(9):257.
24. Heubner O. Tumor der glandula pinealis. Dtsch Med Wochenschr 1898;24:214.
25. Marburg O. Zur kenntnis der normalen und pathologischen histologie der zirbeldriise. Arb Wien Neurol Inst 1907;17:217–49.
26. Marburg O. Die Adipositas cerebralis. Wien Med Wochenschr 1908;2:2617–22.
27. Marburg O. Die physiologie der zirbeldriise (glandula pinealis). Handbuch Der Normalen Und Pathologischen Physiologie 1930;13:493–590.
28. Marburg O. Die klinik der zirbeldriisenerkrankung. Ergebn Inn Med 1913;10:146–66.
29. Berblinger W. Zur kenntnis der zirbelgeschwtilste. Z Neurol 1925;95:741–61.
30. Engel P. Die physiologische und pathologisehe Bedeutung der Zirbeldriise. Ergebn Inn Med 1936;50:116–71.
31. Bustamente M. Experimented untersuchungen uber die lcistungen des hypothalamus, besonders bezuglich der geschlcchtsreifung. Arch Psych 1943;115:419–68.
32. Bargmann W. Die Epiphysis cerebri. In: von Mollendorff W, editor. Handbuch der mikroskopischen Anatomie des Menschen, vol. 6. (Berlin): Springer-Verlag; 1943. p. 309–505.
33. Oksche A, Hartwig HG. Pineal sense organs— components of photoneuroendocrine systems. Prog Brain Res 1979;52:113–30.
34. Collin JP. Contribution a l'etude de l'organe pineale. De 1 'epiphyse sensorielle a la glande pine- ale: modalites de transformation et implications fonctionelles. Besseen-Chandesse. Stat Biol 1969;(Suppl 1):1–359.
35. Lerner AB, Case JD, Heinzelman RV. Structure of melatonin. J Am Chem Soc 1959;81:60–84.
36. Lerner AB. Melatonin. J.D. Fed Proc 1960;19:590–3.

37. Borit A. History of tumors of the pineal region. Am J Surg Pathol 1981;5(6):613–20.

38. Axelrod JA, Weissbach H. Enzymatic O-methylation of N-acetylserotonin to melatonin. Science 1960;138:1312.

39. McISAAC WM, Page IH. The metabolism of serotonin (5-hydroxytryptamine). J Biol Chem 1959; 234:858–64.

40. Fiske VM, Bryant GK, Putnam K. Effect of light on the weight of the pineal in the rat. Endocrinology 1960;66:489–91.

41. Fiske VM. Effect of light on sexual maturation, estrous cycles and anterior pituitary of the rat. Endocrinology 1941;29:187–96.

42. Quay WB, aH A. Experimental modification of the rat's pineal content of serotonin and related indole amines. Physiol Zool 1962;1:1–7.

43. Quay WB. Cytologic and metabolic parameters of pineal inhibition by continuous light in the rat (Rattus norvegicus). Z Zellforsch Mikrosk Anat 1963; 60(3):479–90.

44. Quay WB. Reduction of mammalian pineal weight and lipid during continuous light. Gen Comp Endocrinol 1961;1(3):211–7.

45. Fiske VM. Serotonin rhythm in the pineal organ: control by the sympathetic nervous system. Science 1964;146(3641):253–4.

46. Snyder SH, Axelrod J. Circadian rhythm in pineal serotonin: effect of monoamine oxidase inhibition and reserpine. Science 1965;149(3683):542–3.

47. Lynch H, Wurtman R, Moskowitz M, et al. Daily rhythm in human urinary melatonin. Science 1975; 187(4172):169–71.

48. Drelincurtius C, Manget JJ. Theatrum anatomicum. Geneva (Switzerland): Cramer & Perachon; 1717:309.

49. Morgagni G. De sedibus et causis morborum per anatomen indagatis (the seats and causes of diseases by anatomy). Bethesda (MD): Translation, Published by Classics of Medicine Library Futura; 1761. Original in Italian- Tanslation by Alexander.

50. Blane G. Case of a tumor found in the situation of the pineal gland. Trans Soc Improu Med Know 1800;2:198–207.

51. Smollett T. The critical review, or, annals of literature. Simpkin W, Marshall R. editors. London (England): Princeton University; 1801.

52. Good J. The study of medicine. New York (NY): Harper & Brothers; 1864.

53. Pearce JM. Parinaud's syndrome. J Neurol Neurosurg Psychiatr 2005;76(1):99.

54. Weigert C. Zur lehre von den tumoren der hirnanhange. 1. teratom der zirbeldriise. Virchows Arch 1875;65:212–9.

55. Gutzeit RE. Ein teratom der zirbeldriise. Inauguraldissertation der medicinischen facultat zu konigsberg i. pr zur erlangung der doctorwurde. Konisberg Germany; 1896.

56. Heubner. Tumor der glandula pinealis. Dtsch Med Wochenschr 1898;24:214–5.

57. Oestreich R, Slawyk un. Riesenwuchs und zirbel-driisen-geschwulst. Virchows Arch 1899;157:475–84.

58. Frankl-Hochwart L. Über diagnose der zirbcldriisentumoren. Dtsch Z Neruenheilk 1909;37:455–65.

59. Pellizzi GB. La sindrome epifisaria "macrogenitosomia precoce". Riv Ital di Neuropatol, Psichiat, ed Elettroter 1910;3:193–207, 250–72.

60. Neumann M. Zur kenntnis der zirbeldrüsengeschwülste. Mschr Psychiatrie Neurol 1901;9:337–67.

61. Krabbe KH. The pineal gland, especially in relation to the problem on its supposed significance in sexual development. Endocrinology 1923;7(3): 379–414.

62. Horrax G, Bailey P. Tumors of the pineal body. Arch Neurol Psychiatry 1925;13(4):423–70.

63. Bailey P, Cushing H. A classification of the tumors of the glioma group on a histogenetic basis with a correlated study of prognosis. Philadelphia: Lippincott; 1926.

64. Bailey P, Cushing H. Medulloblastoma cerebelli: a common type of midcerebellar glioma of childhood. Arch Neurol Psychiatry 1925;14(2):192–224.

65. Russell DS, Rubinstein LJ. Pathology of tumours of the nervous system. London: Edward Arnold; 1959.

66. Ziilch KJ. Brain tumors. Their biology and pathology. New York: Springer; 1965.

67. Globus JH, Silbert S. Pinealomas. Arch Neurol Psychiatry 1931;25:937–85.

68. Russell DS. The pinealoma: its relationship to teratoma. J Pathol Bacteriol 1944;56:145–50.

69. Friedman NB. Germinoma of the pineal. Its identity with germinoma ("seminoma") of the testis. Cancer Res 1947;7:363–8.

70. Borden ST, Weber AL, Toch R, et al. Pineal germinoma. Long-term survival despite hematogenous metastases. Am J Dis Child 1973;126(2):214–6.

71. Bebin J. Seminar in neuropathology: part III. Germinoma (atypical pineal teratoma, ectopic pinealoma). J Miss State Med Assoc 1974;15(8):329–30.

72. del Rio-Hortega P, Thomas CC, editors. The microscopic anatomy of tumors of the central and peripheral nervous system. Toronto (Ontario): The Ryerson Press; 1933.

73. Dandy WE. Surgery of the brain, a monograph from Vol. XII, Lewis' Practice of surgery. Hagerstown (MD): W. F. Prior Co, Inc; 1945.

74. Bernstein M. Neuro-oncology: the essentials. New York: Thieme; 2007.

75. Victor H. Discussion of paper by CMH Howell on tumors of the pineal body. Proc R Soc Med 1910;3: 77–8.

76. Pendl G. The surgery of pineal lesions—historical perspective. In: AE N, editor. Diagnosis and treatment of pineal region tumors. Baltimore (MD): Williams & Wilkins; 1984. p. 139–54.

77. Brunner CR, Rorschach H. Uber einen fall von tumor der glandula pinealis cerebri. Cor Blatt Schweiz Arzte 1911;642–3.

78. Zulch KJ. Reflections on the surgery of the pineal gland (a glimpse into the past). Gleanings from medical history. Neurosurg Rev 1981;4(3):159–63.

79. Oppenheim H, Krause F. Operative Erfolge bei Geschwiilsten der Sehhügel—und Vierhugelgegend. Bed Klin Wschr 1913;50:2316–22.

80. Schmidek H. Pineal tumors. Philadelphia (PA): Masson Pub; 1977.

81. Dandy WE. Extirpation of the pineal body. J Exp Med 1915;22:237–47.

82. Dandy WE. An operation for the removal of pineal tumors. Surg Gynecol Obstet 1921;33:113–9.

83. Dandy WE. Operative experiences in cases of pineal tumors. Arch Surg 1936;33:19–46.

84. Camins MB, Schlesinger EB. Treatment of tumours of the posterior part of the third ventricle and the pineal region: a long term follow-up. Acta Neurochir 1978;40:131–43.

85. Horrax G. Extirpation of a large pinealoma from a patient with pubertas parecox: a new operative approach. Arch Neurol Psychiatr 1937;37:385–97.

86. Foerster O. Ein fall von vierhfigeltumor durch operation entfernt. Nervenkr. Arch Psychiat 1928;84:515–6.

87. Van Wagenen W. A surgical approach for the removal of certain pineal tumors. Surg Gynecol Obstet 1931;53:216–20.

88. Rand RW, Lemmen LJ. Tumors of the posterior portion of the third ventricle. J Neurosurg 1953;10(1):1–18.

89. Ringertz N, Nordenstam H, Flyger G. Tumors of the pineal region. J Neuropathol Exp Neurol 1954;13(4):540–61.

90. Poppen JL, Marino R Jr. Pinealomas and tumors of the posterior portion of the third ventricle. J Neurosurg 1968;28(4):357–64.

91. Ward A, Spurling RG. The conservative treatment of third ventricle tumors. J Neurosurg 1948;5(2):124–30.

92. Torkildsen A. Should extirpation be attempted in cases of neoplasm in or near the third ventricle of the brain? experiences with a palliative method. J Neurosurg 1948;5(3):249–75.

93. Lekovic GP, Gonzalez LF, Shetter AG, et al. Role of gamma knife surgery in the management of pineal region tumors. Neurosurg Focus 2007;23(6):E12.

94. Zapletal B. [Surgical approach to the region of incisura tentorii]. Zentralbl Neurochir 1956;16(2):64–9.

95. Stein BM. The infratentorial supracerebellar approach to pineal lesions. J Neurosurg 1971;35(2):197–202.

96. Isamat F. Tumours of the posterior part of the third ventricle: neurosurgical criteria, vol. 6. New York: Springer-Verlag; 1979.

97. Kobayashi S, Sugita K, Tanaka Y, et al. Infratentorial approach to the pineal region in the prone position: concorde position. J Neurosurg 1983;58(1):141–3.

98. Lazar ML, Clark K. Direct surgical management of masses in the region of the vein of galen. Surg Neurol 1974;2(1):17–21.

99. Neuwelt EA, Glasberg M, Frenkel E, et al. Malignant pineal region tumors. A clinico-pathological study. J Neurosurg 1979;51(5):597–607.

100. Page LK. The infratentorial-supracerebellar exposure of tumors in the pineal area. Neurosurgery 1977;1(1):36–40.

101. Reid WS, Clark WK. Comparison of the infratentorial and transtentorial approaches to the pineal region. Neurosurgery 1978;3(1):1–8.

102. Rozario R, Adelman L, Prager RJ, et al. Meningiomas of the pineal region and third ventricle. Neurosurgery 1979;5(4):489–95.

103. Gangemi M, Maiuri F, Colella G, et al. Endoscopic surgery for pineal region tumors. Minim Invasive Neurosurg 2001;44(2):70–3.

104. Alexander NK, David IP. Principles of treatment of the pineal region tumors. Surg Neurol 2003;59(4):252–70.

105. Oi S, Shibata M, Tominaga J, et al. Efficacy of neuroendoscopic procedures in minimally invasive preferential management of pineal region tumors: a prospective study. J Neurosurg 2000;93(2):245–53.

106. Fukushima T, Ishijima B, Hirakawa K, et al. Ventriculofiberscope: a new technique for endoscopic diagnosis and operation. Technical note. J Neurosurg 1973;38(2):251–6.

107. Morgenstern PF, Osbun N, Schwartz TH, et al. Pineal region tumors: an optimal approach for simultaneous endoscopic third ventriculostomy and biopsy. Neurosurg Focus 2011;30(4):E3.

108. Yamini B, Refai D, Rubin CM, et al. Initial endoscopic management of pineal region tumors and associated hydrocephalus: clinical series and literature review. J Neurosurg 2004;100(Suppl 5 Pediatrics):437–41.

109. Robinson S, Cohen AR. The role of neuroendoscopy in the treatment of pineal region tumors. Surg Neurol 1997;48(4):360–5 [discussion: 365–7].

Pathology of Pineal Parenchymal Tumors

Seunggu J. Han, MD[a], Aaron J. Clark, MD, PhD[a],
Michael E. Ivan, MD[a], Andrew T. Parsa, MD, PhD[a],*,
Arie Perry, MD[a,b]

KEYWORDS

- Pineal parenchymal tumors
- Pineocytomas • Pineoblastomas
- Pineal parenchymal tumors of intermediate determination

Neoplasms of the pineal region are a rare group of tumors accounting for less than 1% of all intracranial tumors,[1–3] and represent a very clinically and pathologically heterogeneous group of tumors including pineal parenchymal tumors, germ cell tumors, astrocytomas, ependymomas, and papillary pineal tumors. Many investigators have therefore stressed the importance of a tissue-based diagnosis for patient management.[2] Tumors thought to arise from the parenchymal cells of the pineal gland, also referred to as pineal parenchymal tumors, consist of approximately one-third of all tumors of the pineal region.[1,4] The latest World Health Organization (WHO) classification scheme, released in 2007, categorizes pineal parenchymal tumors into 3 subtypes with up to 4 different grade categories: (1) WHO Grade I pineocytomas, (2) WHO Grade II or III pineal parenchymal tumors of intermediate differentiation, and (3) WHO Grade IV pineoblastomas.[5] This review focuses on the spectrum of pathologic features found in these pineal parenchymal tumors.

PINEOCYTOMAS

Pineocytomas are the lowest grade (WHO Grade I) tumors with the most favorable prognosis.[6,7] The 5-year survival has been reported to range from 64% to 91%,[1,8–10] although the latter figure is probably more accurate when strictly defined using the most current criteria. These tumors are found most commonly in the adult population, and clinically appear to progress slowly, although symptomatic recurrences have commonly been reported even after aggressive resection.[11–13] Pineocytomas grossly are well circumscribed and cause symptoms by local growth with local compressive mass effect.[1,8,14]

The histologic features of pineocytomas include their cellular resemblance to mature pineocytes, and they are primarily composed of well-differentiated cells.[4] However, in contrast to the normal pineal gland's lobular architecture created by gliovascular septae (**Fig. 1**A), pineocytomas are arranged in sheets of rounded tumor cells with variable oligodendroglioma-like clear haloes (**Fig. 1**B). Portions of the tumor are occasionally found to have focal ganglionic and/or astrocytic differentiation, and at times cells displaying features of ganglion cells and astrocytes can be found within the same tumor.[11,15] Early studies have suggested a more benign clinical course for pineocytomas with neuronal or neuronal and astrocytic differentiation, with a greater tendency to remain localized as compared with pineocytomas with astrocytic differentiation.[15] More recent studies, however, have failed to establish this correlation.[16] Pineocytomatous rosettes (**Fig. 1**C), also referred to as pineocytic rosettes, are frequently observed, and are believed to be a distinct feature of pineocytomas.[8,11] These rosettes consist of tumor cells surrounding pink neuropil (collections of neuronal processes) and are similar in appearance to

[a] Department of Neurological Surgery, University of California, San Francisco, 505 Parnassus Avenue, M779, Box 0112, San Francisco, CA 94117, USA
[b] Department of Pathology, University of California, San Francisco, 505 Parnassus Avenue, San Francisco, CA 94117, USA
* Corresponding author.
E-mail address: ParsaA@neurosurg.ucsf.edu

Neurosurg Clin N Am 22 (2011) 335–340
doi:10.1016/j.nec.2011.05.006
1042-3680/11/$ – see front matter © 2011 Published by Elsevier Inc.

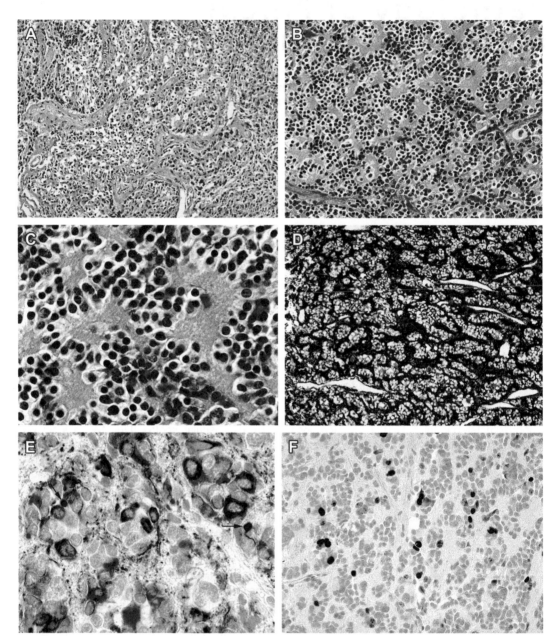

Fig. 1. Comparison of normal pineal gland (*A*) and pineocytoma (*B–F*). The cellularity of normal pineal is surprisingly similar to neoplasms, but the vaguely lobulated architecture created by gliovascular septae is typical of non-neoplastic pineal (*A*). By contrast, pineocytomas often display a sheet-like arrangement of rounded nuclei with variable clear haloes reminiscent of oligodendroglioma (hematoxylin-eosin, original magnification ×100) (*B*). Pineocytomatous rosettes contain central neuropil (pink aggregates of neuronal processes), consistent with a neuronal rather than glial neoplasm (H&E, original magnification ×200) (*C*). This is confirmed immunohistochemically with diffuse synaptophysin (H&E, original magnification ×400) (*D*) and patchy neurofilament (*E*) positivity, the latter sometimes showing bulbous axonal swellings characteristic of pineal differentiation (*E; arrows*) (*D*: Synaptophysin stain, original magnification ×400; *E*: Neurofilament stain, original magnification ×400). The MIB-1 proliferative index is low (*F*) (MIB-1 stain, ×200).

Homer-Wright rosettes, but are formed by mature rather than primitive cells and tend to be somewhat larger and more irregular.[8,17] Despite the occasional resemblance to oligodendrogliomas,

neuronal differentiation is evident in the form of diffuse synaptophysin immunoreactivity (**Fig. 1D**) and often strong positivity for neurofilament protein (**Fig. 1E**), the latter occasionally highlighting bulbous axonal swellings typical of pineal differentiation (arrows in **Fig. 1**E). The level of proliferative activity is relatively low in pineocytomas, with mitoses being rare and MIB-1 (Ki-67) labeling indices averaging around 1.6% (**Fig. 1**F) (the MIB-1 labeling index is the fraction of tumor cells that is labeled by Ki-67).[18,19] In one study, the MIB-1 labeling index was significantly different for each of the 3 pineal parenchymal tumors, and the investigators suggest its use as an additional measure to differentiate between the 3 subtypes.[18]

Cytogenetic studies of pineocytomas have revealed high expression of genes related to phototransduction of the retina (OPN4, RGS16, and CRB3), as well as those related to biosynthesis of melatonin (TPH and HIOMT).[20] Alterations in chromosomes X, 1, 5, 11, and 22 have been demonstrated in karyotypes from pineocytomas,[17,21,22] but on comparative genomic hybridization analysis chromosomal changes were uncommon, with most samples having no such changes.[19]

PINEAL PARENCHYMAL TUMORS OF INTERMEDIATE DIFFERENTIATION

Pineal parenchymal tumors of intermediate differentiation (PPTID) share some features with both pineocytomas and pineoblastomas, but generally lack the more definitive diagnostic features that define these two extremes.[23] The addition of this third intermediate group of tumors in between the two ends of the spectrum of degree of cellular differentiation was proposed by Schild and colleagues[9] in 1993.

At present no definite criteria exist for PPTIDs, but the tumor cells generally have moderate nuclear atypia, mitotic counts are higher (0–16 per 10 high-power fields [HPF]) than pineocytomas, and pineocytic rosettes are inconspicuous, consistent with a partial loss of differentiation.[8] Accordingly, the MIB-1 labeling index is generally higher than in pineocytomas, ranging from 8% to 11.8%.[19,24] Less common features include endothelial hyperplasia and necrosis, but PPTIDs lack the primitive small round cell appearance seen in pineoblastomas. Morphologically, PPTIDs exist in 3 separate subtypes, including (1) the endocrine-like subtype with lobulated growth pattern and increased vascularity (**Fig. 2**A), (2) the oligodendroglioma/neurocytoma-like type with diffuse growth patterns, and (3) transitional type with areas of lobulated and/or diffuse growth patterns intermixed with focal pineocytoma-like regions containing well-formed pineoctyomatous rosettes.[1,8] Multiple studies have noted the impact of the range of histologic features found in pineal parenchymal tumors, even within PPTIDs, on the prognosis of the patients.[1,4,6] In

a study by Jouvet and colleagues,[6] the investigators proposed a new system dividing PPTIDs into two subgroups based on their histology. Low-grade PPTIDs, representing WHO Grade II, can have any of the 3 growth patterns described (transitional, lobulated, or diffuse), and have high expression of neurofilament, similar to pineocytomas.[25,26] The low-grade PPTIDs also have 0 to 5 mitoses per 10 HPF (**Fig. 2**B), with moderate MIB-1 indices (**Fig. 2**C). High-grade PPTIDs are WHO Grade III, do not contain any pineocytoma-like regions, and hence have lobulated or diffuse growth patterns with very limited neurofilament expression, reflecting a more limited degree of neuronal differentiation in comparison with lower-grade examples. The mitotic index is also higher, with typically more than 5 mitoses per 10 HPF encountered, and high MIB-1 labeling indices (**Fig. 2**D). Vascular proliferation and necrosis are also more commonly found in high-grade PPTIDs.

Cytogenetically, PPTIDs have more chromosomal changes, with averages of 5.3 changes (3.3 gains and 2.0 losses) in one study.[19] The most common alterations were gains of 4q and 12q, as well as losses of 22. Commonly overexpressed genes included PRAME, CD24, POU4F2, and HOXD13, with higher levels of expression of each of these genes found in Grade III PPTIDs. Of note, a recent study has also reported expression of the epidermal growth factor receptor variant III in a case of PPTID[27]; however, this finding is yet to be reported by other groups.

As mentioned earlier, the prognosis of patients with PPTID varies by the tumors' histopathologic feature, and hence serves as the basis for the different WHO grades. The 5-year survival rates have been estimated at 74% for Grade II PPTIDs and 39% for Grade III PPTIDs. Similarly, relapse rates are reportedly higher in the Grade III PPTIDs, and progression to pineoblastoma has been reported rarely at recurrence, although this concept remains controversial.[1,28]

PINEOBLASTOMAS

Pineoblastomas are frankly malignant, WHO Grade IV tumors. In some series they represent the most common type of pineal parenchymal tumors, with reported rates of up to half of all pineal parenchymal tumors.[1,9] These blastomas are essentially primitive small round cell tumors that resemble medulloblastomas (**Fig. 3**) that occur primarily in children or infants, with a strong potential for leptomeningeal seeding.[11] Similar to central nervous system primitive neuroectodermal tumors, the prognosis for patients with pineoblastomas is very poor, with 5-year survival rates of only 10%.[1,29]

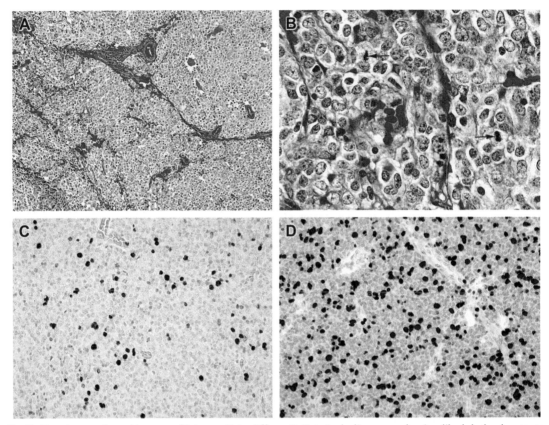

Fig. 2. Pineal parenchymal tumors of intermediate differentiation, including an endocrine-like lobular, hypervascular pattern (*A*) and increased cell size with atypia and scattered mitotic figures (*B*; *arrows*). MIB-1 labeling indices are often moderate in WHO grade II (*C*) and high in WHO grade III (*D*) examples (*A*: H&E, ×100; *B*: H&E, ×200; *C, D*: MIB-1 stain, ×200).

Morphologically, pineoblastomas may have ill-defined borders and grow invasively into surrounding tissue.[30] The tumor shows marked hypercellularity with variable growth patterns, along with variable degrees of necrosis (see **Fig. 3**A).[8] Individual tumor cells contain minimal cytoplasm with high nuclear-cytoplasmic ratios and frequent mitotic figures (see **Fig. 3**B). The tumors may contain Homer-Wright rosettes with central neuropil.[11] Focal expression of neuronal markers is usually present, and there is also variable focal positivity for glial fibrillary acidic protein.[8] The average MIB-1

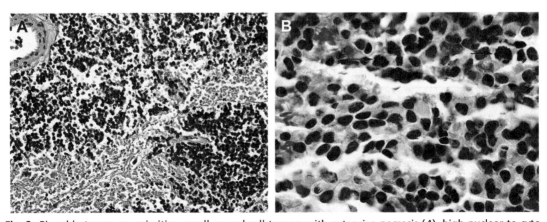

Fig. 3. Pineoblastomas are primitive, small, round cell tumors with extensive necrosis (*A*), high nuclear to cytoplasmic ratios, and high mitotic indices (*B*; *arrows*) (*A*: H&E, ×200; *B*: H&E, ×400).

labeling index is significantly higher in pineoblastomas than in other pineal parenchymal tumors, with average values of 24% to 27%.[18,19,31]

Pineoblastomas frequently have high expression levels of several genes, including *UBEC2*, *SOX4*, *TERT*, *TEP1*, *PRAME*, *CD24*, *POU4F2*, and *HOXD13*.[20,32] Pineoblastomas also frequently exhibit chromosomal imbalances, with averages of 2 to 3 gains and 3 to 4 losses.[19] The most commonly reported chromosomal change was the loss of chromosome 22, but gains of 1, 5, 6, and 14, and loss of 11 were also noted.[19,33]

REFERENCES

1. Fauchon F, Jouvet A, Paquis P, et al. Parenchymal pineal tumors: a clinicopathological study of 76 cases. Int J Radiat Oncol Biol Phys 2000;46(4):959–68.
2. Prahlow JA, Challa VR. Neoplasms of the pineal region. South Med J 1996;89(11):1081–7.
3. Schulte FJ, Herrmann HD, Muller D, et al. Pineal region tumours of childhood. Eur J Pediatr 1987; 146(3):233–45.
4. Linggood RM, Chapman PH. Pineal tumors. J Neurooncol 1992;12(1):85–91.
5. Louis D, Ohgaki H, Wiestler OD, et al. WHO classification of tumors of the central nervous system. World Health Organization classification of tumours. Lyon (France): IARC Press; 2007. p. 122–9.
6. Jouvet A, Saint-Pierre G, Fauchon F, et al. Pineal parenchymal tumors: a correlation of histological features with prognosis in 66 cases. Brain Pathol 2000;10(1):49–60.
7. Deshmukh VR, Smith KA, Rekate HL, et al. Diagnosis and management of pineocytomas. Neurosurgery 2004;55(2):349–55 [discussion: 355–7].
8. Dahiya S, Perry A. Pineal tumors. Adv Anat Pathol 2010;17(6):419–27.
9. Schild SE, Scheithauer BW, Schomberg PJ, et al. Pineal parenchymal tumors. Clinical, pathologic, and therapeutic aspects. Cancer 1993;72(3):870–80.
10. Clark AJ, Sughrue ME, Ivan ME, et al. Factors influencing overall survival rates for patients with pineocytoma. J Neurooncol 2010;100(2):255–60.
11. Borit A, Blackwood W, Mair WG. The separation of pineocytoma from pineoblastoma. Cancer 1980; 45(6):1408–18.
12. Disclafani A, Hudgins RJ, Edwards MS, et al. Pineocytomas. Cancer 1989;63(2):302–4.
13. Tracy PT, Hanigan WC, Kalyan-Raman UP. Radiological and pathological findings in three cases of childhood pineocytomas. Childs Nerv Syst 1986;2(6): 297–300.
14. Schild SE, Scheithauer BW, Haddock MG, et al. Histologically confirmed pineal tumors and other germ cell tumors of the brain. Cancer 1996;78(12): 2564–71.
15. Herrick MK, Rubinstein LJ. The cytological differentiating potential of pineal parenchymal neoplasms (true pinealomas). A clinicopathological study of 28 tumours. Brain 1979;102(2):289–320.
16. Mena H, Rushing EJ, Ribas JL, et al. Tumors of pineal parenchymal cells: a correlation of histological features, including nucleolar organizer regions, with survival in 35 cases. Hum Pathol 1995;26(1): 20–30.
17. Dario A, Cerati M, Taborelli M, et al. Cytogenetic and ultrastructural study of a pineocytoma case report. J Neurooncol 2000;48(2):131–4.
18. Arivazhagan A, Anandh B, Santosh V, et al. Pineal parenchymal tumors—utility of immunohistochemical markers in prognostication. Clin Neuropathol 2008;27(5):325–33.
19. Rickert CH, Simon R, Bergmann M, et al. Comparative genomic hybridization in pineal parenchymal tumors. Genes Chromosomes Cancer 2001;30(1): 99–104.
20. Fevre-Montange M, Champier J, Szathmari A, et al. Microarray analysis reveals differential gene expression patterns in tumors of the pineal region. J Neuropathol Exp Neurol 2006;65(7):675–84.
21. Bello MJ, Rey JA, de Campos JM, et al. Chromosomal abnormalities in a pineocytoma. Cancer Genet Cytogenet 1993;71(2):185–6.
22. Rainho CA, Rogatto SR, de Moraes LC, et al. Cytogenetic study of a pineocytoma. Cancer Genet Cytogenet 1992;64(2):127–32.
23. Sato K, Kubota T. Pathology of pineal parenchymal tumors. Prog Neurol Surg 2009;23:12–25.
24. Fevre-Montange M, Szathmari A, Champier J, et al. Pineocytoma and pineal parenchymal tumors of intermediate differentiation presenting cytologic pleomorphism: a multicenter study. Brain Pathol 2008;18(3): 354–9.
25. Sasaki A, Horiguchi K, Nakazato Y. Pineal parenchymal tumor of intermediate differentiation with cytologic pleomorphism. Neuropathology 2006; 26(3):212–7.
26. Pusztaszeri M, Pica A, Janzer R. Pineal parenchymal tumors of intermediate differentiation in adults: case report and literature review. Neuropathology 2006;26(2):153–7.
27. Li G, Mitra S, Karamchandani J, et al. Pineal parenchymal tumor of intermediate differentiation: clinicopathological report and analysis of epidermal growth factor receptor variant III expression. Neurosurgery 2010;66(5):963–8 [discussion: 968].
28. Kim BS, Kim DK, Park SH. Pineal parenchymal tumor of intermediate differentiation showing malignant progression at relapse. Neuropathology 2009; 29(5):602–8.
29. Al-Hussaini M, Sultan I, Abuirmileh N, et al. Pineal gland tumors: experience from the SEER database. J Neurooncol 2009;94(3):351–8.

30. Chang SM, Lillis-Hearne PK, Larson DA, et al. Pineoblastoma in adults. Neurosurgery 1995;37(3):383–90 [discussion: 390–1].

31. Tsumanuma I, Tanaka R, Washiyama K. Clinicopathological study of pineal parenchymal tumors: correlation between histopathological features, proliferative potential, and prognosis. Brain Tumor Pathol 1999;16(2):61–8.

32. Fevre-Montange M, Vasiljevic A, Champier J, et al. Histopathology of tumors of the pineal region. Future Oncol 2010;6(5):791–809.

33. Sreekantaiah C, Jockin H, Brecher ML, et al. Interstitial deletion of chromosome 11q in a pineoblastoma. Cancer Genet Cytogenet 1989;39(1): 125–31.

Pineal Cyst: A Review of Clinical and Radiological Features

Winward Choy, BA, Won Kim, MD, Marko Spasic, BA, Brittany Voth, BS, Andrew Yew, MD, Isaac Yang, MD*

KEYWORDS

- Pineal cysts • Imaging modality • Pineal region
- Radiographic features

Pineal cysts (PCs) are benign and often asymptomatic lesions of the pineal region found in 33% to 40% of autopsy series.[1–3] Several retrospective studies have reported incidences of PCs that range from 1.5% to 10.8%.[2,4–10] Incidence is higher in females than in males, is greatest between the ages of 21 and 30 years, and decreases with increasing age.[11] Overall, females between 21 and 30 years of age have the greatest frequency at 5.82%.[11]

The precise etiology of PCs remains unclear, and several investigators have suggested several theories explaining PC pathogenesis.[11–14] During development, the walls of the third ventricle diverticulum proliferate to form the pineal gland. During this process, remnants of the diverticulum may form a cavity lined with cells that can differentiate into ependymal cells. PCs with an ependymal lining may consequently result from an enlargement of the embryonic pineal cavity.[15] However, some PCs are not lined with ependymal cells, but are rather surrounded by a glial scar.[16,17] This observation has led some investigators to believe that PCs can arise from ischemic degeneration of glial plaques. Others have suggested that PCs result from necrotic pineal parenchyma; however, the cause of the necrosis is unclear.[16,17]

While these hypotheses may account for the pathogenesis of smaller cysts, the mechanisms underlying the formation of larger and symptomatic cysts have yet to be elucidated.[1,11] Findings of microscopic cysts in autopsy series have led some investigators to believe that larger cysts may arise when smaller cysts coalesce to form larger lesions.[16,18] However, given the stagnancy of growth in reports examining the natural history of PCs, this hypothesis is unlikely.[16,18,19] Other investigators noting the presence of hemosiderin intraoperatively have suggested that cysts may form through hemorrhage.[16–18,20,21] Klein and Rubinstein[18] have suggested that the large female preponderance of PCs, particularly at younger ages during onset of puberty with decrease in incidence with older age, is suggestive of a hormonal influence on PC development.[11,18] Indeed, a female prevalence has been noted in several studies,[11,16,18,19,22] which could be explained by a hormonal component associated with the menstrual cycle or pregnancy.[11,16–18]

CLINICAL FEATURES

The majority of pineal cysts are small, and roughly 80% of cysts are less than 10 mm in diameter.[15] Cysts smaller than 10 mm in diameter are often asymptomatic,[23] and larger cysts (diameter >15 mm) may lead to neurologic symptoms resulting from local mass effect on adjacent structures or hydrocephalus through compression of the aqueduct.[15,24] Increased frequency and improved resolution of neuroimaging technologies and contrast administration have led to an increase in the detection of incidental PCs.[7,8,25–27] Symptomatic lesions are often larger than those found

Department of Neurological Surgery, University of California, Los Angeles, 695 Charles E Young Drive South, Gonda 3357, Los Angeles, CA 90095-1761, USA
* Corresponding author.
E-mail address: iyang@mednet.ucla.edu

Neurosurg Clin N Am 22 (2011) 341–351
doi:10.1016/j.nec.2011.06.001
1042-3680/11/$ – see front matter © 2011 Elsevier Inc. All rights reserved.

incidentally, and occur most often in women in their second decade of life.[11,28]

Histologically, PCs are composed of 3 distinct layers. The inner layer comprises fibrillar glial tissue, with or without hemosiderin, and is surrounded by a middle layer of pineal parenchymal tissue that can contain calcium deposits. The outermost layer is a thin layer of leptomeningeal fibrous tissue.[15] During surgery, PCs appear smooth and unilocular with a tan outer layer. Cystic contents are variable and may contain watery, hemorrhagic, or coagulated fluid,[11,17–19] and other reports have found that cyst contents can have elevated protein levels.[5,7,8]

The natural course of PCs is typically benign, and several studies have found that PCs rarely change in size over time.[29] Golzarian and colleagues[5] found no detectable change in cyst size on magnetic resonance imaging (MRI) scans in 12 patients with follow-up longer than 1 year. Tamaki and colleagues[25] reported on 31 patients with PCs with a follow-up ranging from 3 months to 4 years, and found stable disease except for a decrease in cyst size in 2 patients. In a study of 32 patients with a mean follow-up of 3.7 years (range 6 months to 9 years), Barboriak and colleagues[24] found no change in cyst size in 75% of patients. Cysts completely resolved in 2 patients and decreased by 2 to 4 mm in 3 others. Cysts in 2 patients increased in size, and one patient had a newly formed cyst that was 12 mm in diameter. No correlation was found between changes in cyst size over the course of the study and follow-up duration, cyst size at initial diagnosis, or age. Recently, Al-Holou and colleagues[30] reported a study of 106 young patients (<25 years old) with PCs and an average follow-up of 3 years. On follow-up MRI scans, 98 PCs (92%) did not change in size or imaging characteristics. Six PCs increased in size by an average of 4.4 mm in diameter, and 1 decreased in size. In addition, a change in cyst appearance on MRI, either the development of a posterior enhancing nodule or novel separations was noted in 4 cysts. Similar to previous findings, the vast majority of cysts do not change in size or appearance over time, and the initial cyst size, appearance on MRI, sex, and change in symptoms were not correlated with PC growth during later follow-up.

Given the high number of benign PCs found incidentally through MRI and the largely stagnant natural history of these asymptomatic PCs, it is unrealistic to follow up every patient. Rather, investigators have suggested periodic follow-up in patients with cysts that have abnormal imaging characteristics,[24,31] in younger patients,[30] and in patients with cysts larger than 10 mm.[24] However,

there has not been clear evidence suggesting that larger cysts or cysts with atypical imaging features are particularly prone to change in size or become symptomatic.[24] Increases in cyst size in asymptomatic patients have not been associated with the development of symptoms. Lastly, studies have found that cysts greater than 5 mm in diameter are rare in elderly patients[1,11,25] and also in patients younger than 10 years.[25] It is possible that in asymptomatic cysts, small growth, particularly through adulthood, may merely reflect a benign and natural cyst growth and involution pattern not indicative of symptom development.[24] Thus, several studies have suggested against interval imaging follow-ups for patients with PCs smaller than 14 mm.[24,32,33]

SYMPTOMS

Symptomatic pineal cysts are rare and, consequently, reports have been rare as well.[17,19,22,34] Most pineal cysts are found incidentally, and are asymptomatic and independent of initial presenting symptoms.[6] Even when there is growth in an initially asymptomatic PC, the lesion is likely to remain asymptomatic.[30] However, when symptoms do develop, clinical manifestations of PCs and other pineal pathologies are intimately tied to the unique location and physiology of the pineal gland.

Pinocytes, the main parenchymal cell within the pineal gland, link sympathetic input from the retina to the production of melatonin, which is involved in the regulation of wake-sleep cycles and the release of other hormones.[35,36] However, it is unclear as to what extent the presence of PCs alter the regular production and secretion of these hormones.[6] Significant compromise of pineal gland function may lead to irregular melatonin production and be subsequent to hormonal imbalance. Precocious puberty is one of the more common endocrine imbalances associated with PCs,[37] and rarer symptoms reported include hypogonadism and diabetes insipidus.[38]

Given the sensitive location of the pineal gland, even small masses may have potentially serious consequences. Cerebellar, corticospinal, and sensory disturbances may result from direct compression of the midbrain.[18] If large enough, PCs can lead to hydrocephalus associated with aqueductal compression, blockage of the vein of Galen, and symptoms of raised intracranial pressure.[28] Compression of the superior colliculus leads to Parinaud syndrome, characterized by number of abnormalities in eye movement and pupillary function including upgaze palsy, light-near dissociation of pupils, and convergence-retraction nystagmus.[20]

Headaches are the most common neurologic symptom of patients with pineal cysts.[39] In a case-control study examining the association between headaches and pineal cysts, Seifert and colleagues[35] found that patients with PC were twice as likely to develop headaches when compared with age-matched and sex-matched controls (51% vs 25%) and that the most frequent presenting symptom was migraines (26%). Of the 51 patients with PCs, 14% presented with migraine with aura, whereas only 2% of the patients in the control group had migraines with aura. While there have been some reports that large benign cysts can lead to hydrocephalus resulting in headache,[40–42] many investigators suggest that the mechanisms producing headaches in patients with PCs are not associated with compression or mass effect.[39,40] In support of this, many patients with PCs exhibiting compression of the quadrigeminal lamina as determined by MRI are asymptomatic.[40] The observation that none of these patients had hydrocephalus and that size of the PC did not vary between patients with and without headaches in the study by Seifert and colleagues[35] led the investigators to propose a possible role of abnormal melatonin production, rather than mass effect, to be responsible for the reported headaches. Evidence from other studies has demonstrated a link between headache disorders and melatonin,[28,43–48] but the precise mechanisms underlying the association with PCs are still unclear.

Other less common nonspecific signs include seizures, headaches, vertigo, blurred vision, hemiparesis, and vomiting.[29,49,50] Rarer complications that have been reported include pineal apoplexy resulting from intracystic hemorrhage,[2,51,52] development of secondary parkinsonian symptoms (eg, resting tremor),[53] development of choroid plexus papilloma,[31] and aseptic meningitis from cyst rupture.[29,54]

RADIOLOGICAL FEATURES

PCs appear as small, adequately circumscribed, unilocular masses within the pineal gland typically measuring less than 10 mm in diameter. Cysts can range from 5 to 15 mm in many asymptomatic patients and can also be as large as 45 mm in diameter in symptomatic cases.[4,17,25,41,55] PCs can either reside within or completely replace the pineal gland.[56] Signal intensity is variable and is dependent on the cystic components.[15] In addition, PCs typically do not exhibit compression of adjacent structures including the cerebral aqueduct, vein of Galen, and the quadrigeminal plate.[57]

Computed Tomography

On computed tomography (CT), PCs can appear hypodense relative to cerebrospinal fluid (CSF)[17,25,28] (**Fig. 1**). Regions or nodules of hyperdensity may be detected because of hemorrhage or calcification.[21,58] Roughly 25% to 33% of PCs may contain thin rim calcifications along cyst walls.[17,23,28] However, the contents of the PC can be either homogeneous or heterogeneous, and may have either a unilocular or polycystic appearance.[58,59] On contrast imaging, PCs exhibit contrast enhancement peripherally.[23] Some investigators have noted that smaller pineal cysts are not clearly detectable on CT and should require further MRI for confirmation.[17] In a retrospective study by Tamaki and colleagues,[25] 32 patients with PCs received initial CT scans. A low-density mass diagnostic of a PC was found

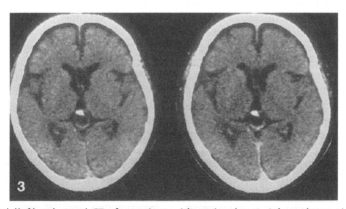

Fig. 1. (*Right*) CT and (*left*) enhanced CT of a patient with a pineal cyst. A hypodense pineal cyst along with a posterior nodule and anterior dots of calcification are seen. (*Reprinted from* Tamaki N, Shirataki K, Lin TK, et al. Cysts of the pineal gland. A new clinical entity to be distinguished from tumors of the pineal region. Childs Nerv Syst 1989;5:173. Copyright 1989; with permission from Springer.)

in 12 patients (37.5%). In addition, CT imaging revealed slight dotted or nodular sharply enhancing calcifications along the cyst walls.[18,25,41,55] However, in the remaining 20 patients (63%), CT imaging did not identify the PCs, and additional imaging was required. Similarly, Fain and colleagues[17] found calcification in only 3 of 9 patients (33%) through CT. This failure to show PCs on CT scans is likely due to the similar densities of CSF and PCs.[25]

Magnetic Resonance Imaging

On MRI, PCs are sharply defined ovoid lesions with smooth margins (**Fig. 2**).[5,6,8,20,56] The contents of PCs are homogeneous and lack intracystic trabeculations. Because cystic contents are typically aqueous or contain protein, PCs usually have signal characteristics similar to CSF.[7,23,28] Several studies using traditional MRI techniques to examine PCs have reported their configurations and imaging characteristics.[5,7,8,11,17,19,25,41]

In one of the earlier retrospective MR studies of PCs, Lee and colleagues[7] reviewed 1000 MR scans and identified 15 patients with PCs. The majority of cases were incidental findings on routine MRI. Patients were scanned with either a 1.5-T or 0.35-T imaging unit. Mean age was 30 years, and cyst diameters ranged from 5 to 15 mm. On imaging, PCs often had smooth borders with homogeneous cystic contents. On T1-weighted imaging (T1-WI), 11 out of 15 (73.3%) showed slightly increased signaling intensity, and the remaining 4 (26%) were isointense relative to CSF in adjacent ventricles. On T2-weighted imaging (T2-WI), 10 (66.7%) showed markedly increased signaling intensity, 3 (20%) were slightly increased, 1 (6.7%) was isointense, and 1 (6.7%) was hyperintense relative to CSF. The cyst walls were thin and ranged from 1.0 to 2.0 mm, and there was no evidence of compression of the third ventricle or collicular plates, or hydrocephalus.

Jinkins and colleagues[6] reported the imaging characteristics of 60 patients with PCs. Most cysts appeared unilocular while 2 (3.3%) showed septations. On T1-WI (repetition time/echo time 500/20 ms, thickness 5 mm), 37 (62%) were hyperintense, 17 (28%) were isointense, and 6 (10%) were hypointense. On proton-density–weighted imaging (PD-WI) (2400/30 ms, 5 mm), 43 (72%) were hyperintense, 14 (23%) were isointense, and 2 (5%) were hypointense. Finally, on T2-WI (2400/80 ms, 5 mm), 23 (38%) were hyperintense, 34 (57%) were isointense, and 3 (5%) were hypointense. All patients receiving T1-WI immediately following intravenous (IV) administration of gadolinium showed a thin rim of enhancement. In addition, in 2 patients receiving IV gadolinium following delay of up to 60 minutes, T1-WI showed central enhancement of the lesion (**Fig. 3**). Thinning of the superior colliculi of the quadrigeminal plate was observed in 19 patients (32%), and no hydrocephalus was detected in any patient.

Barboriak and colleagues[24] reported similar findings in a retrospective study analyzing the natural history of typical PCs that compared MR images taken initially at diagnosis and those taken most recently with a minimum of 6 months follow-up. All images were obtained with a 1.5-T imaging unit. Typical PCs are defined as those that are (1) lesion(s) centered in the pineal recess with smooth, regular margins, (2) hypointense to white matter on T1-WI and isointense with CSF on T2-WI, and (3) homogeneous cystic components on T2-WI. In total, 32 (71.1%) patients satisfied inclusion criteria. The average cyst diameter and volume was 11.2 mm and 1.42 cm³, respectively. On PD-WI, 88% of cysts were hyperintense, and 12% were isointense to CSF. There were variable grades of tectal deformity resulting from the mass effect of the PC, with 32% of scans exhibiting some extent of tectal deformity and one patient exhibiting severe tectal deformity and aqueductal narrowing. None of the cysts showed nodular enhancement on either the initial or the final scans.

In the largest study to date on PCs, Al-Holou and colleagues[16] examined the clinical characteristics of pineal cysts in younger patients. The investigators retrospectively reviewed 14,516 consecutive patients younger than 25 years who had received MRI scans at their institution. Either a 1.5-T or 3-T MRI unit was used in the scans reviewed, and only PCs with a diameter equal to or greater than 5 mm were included. "Normal" radiological features were defined as having homogeneous cystic contents, being isointense or slightly hyperintense on both T1-WI and T2-WI, showing a smooth and thin cyst rim measuring less than 2 mm, and lacking an irregular mass or nodularity. The frequency of PCs was 2.0% (n = 288), with a female preponderance of 2.4% (compared with 1.5% of males, P<.001). Detailed imaging was available for 108 of the 288 patients with PCs. Average cyst size was 10.0 ± 4.3 mm sagittal anteroposteriorly, 6.7 ± 2.8 mm sagittal craniocaudal plane, 9.3 ± 4.5 mm axially, and 8.7 ± 2.8 mm coronally. Because most cysts were small, minimal to no compression of the cerebral aqueduct and quadrigeminal plate was found in 95% of cases. On T1-WI 97% of PCs were isointense or slightly hyperintense, and 3% were hyperintense relative to CSF. On T2-WI 97% of PCs were isointense or slightly hyperintense, 1% were hyperintense, and 2% were hypointense relative to CSF. A thin

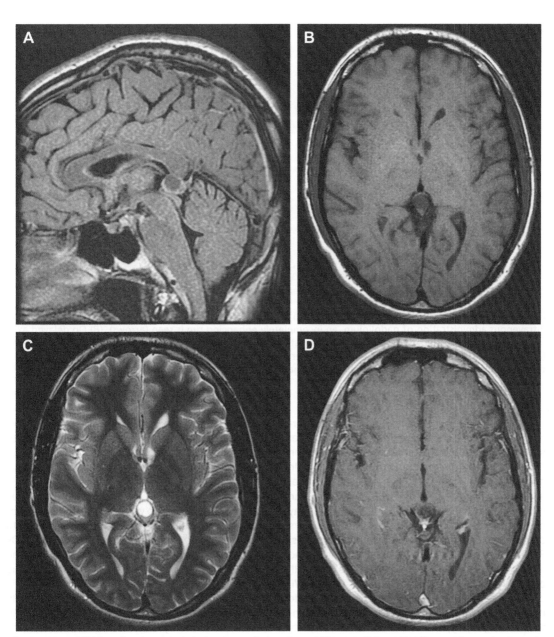

Fig. 2. MRI exhibiting the characteristic features of pineal cysts. The cyst (14 mm in diameter) appears hyperintense with respect to CSF and hypointense relative to white matter on fluid-attenuated inversion recovery (FLAIR) (*A*); is hypointense relative to white matter and either isointense or diffusely hyperintense relative to CSF on T1-weighted images (*B*); and has a homogeneous appearance and is slightly hyperintense relative to CSF on T2-weighted imaging (*C*). Although on contrast-enhanced T1-weighted images cysts typically have a uniformly enhancing rim, an atypical thin nonenhancing rim is seen in this patient (*D*). The hyperintensity of the pineal cyst relative to CSF on FLAIR and T1-weighted images indicates increased protein content. (*Reprinted from* Gaillard F, Jones J. Masses of the pineal region: clinical presentation and radiographic features. Postgrad Med J 2010;86:599. Copyright 2010; with permission from BMJ Publishing Group Ltd.)

rim measuring less than 2 mm was found in 88% of PCs and exhibited enhancement in 92% of cases. Cystic contents were homogeneous in 52%, and normal imaging characteristics were found in 47%. Atypical imaging characteristics were commonly attributed to the presence of septations (22%) and irregular enhancing nodularities (16%) located in the posterior aspect of the cyst. This abnormal enhancement may likely represent a venous structure or a displaced pineal gland.

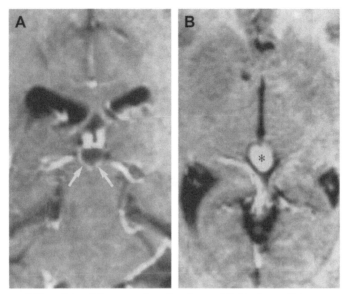

Fig. 3. Contrast-enhanced T1-weighted images of a pineal cyst. (*A*) On immediate coronal imaging following intravenous administration of gadolinium, an incompletely enhancing rim is seen (*arrows*). (*B*) On delayed axial imaging 60 minutes following gadolinium administration, the cavity is completely and uniformly enhancing (*asterisk*). (*Reprinted from* Jinkins JR, Xiong L, Reiter RJ. The midline pineal "eye": MR and CT characteristics of the pineal gland with and without benign cyst formation. J Pineal Res 1995;19:67. Copyright 1995; with permission from John Wiley and Sons.)

Atypical pineal cyst features are not rare occurrences and have been reported in several other studies. The presence of septations is a common radiological finding in numerous patients.[1,16,60] In some reports, scans of PCs, particularly after a delay following contrast administration, can often exhibit abnormal enhancement that may mimic the imaging characteristics of solid tumors of the pineal region.[16,61] In a study of 24 patients, Fain and colleagues[17] reviewed the clinical and radiological characteristics of large PCs. On MRI, cysts were typically homogeneous. On T1-WI, cysts appeared hypointense compared with white matter; whereas on T2-WI, cysts appeared isointense or slightly hyperintense relative to CSF. Fifty percent of patients with MRI scans (6 of 12) had nodular enhancements following intravenous administration of gadolinium. Enhancements were variable in size but commonly appeared, on the sagittal plane, as an enhancing bulb found in the posterior pineal region. The characteristic thin enhancing ring was still visible, encompassing the remaining regions of the pineal cyst. In addition, the investigators found evidence of previous hemorrhage in 18% of patients. Fleege and colleagues[20] reported similar results in another review of 19 patients with histologically confirmed and symptomatic PCs. These symptomatic cysts may be associated with atypical cyst features, including larger diameter (>16 mm), atypical

nodular enhancement (58% of cases), and hemorrhage (18% of cases).[16,20] These nodular enhancements can be attributed to adjacent vascularity[5,16] or the appearance of posteriorly displaced pineal tissue.[16,56]

Overall, on T1-WI PCs appear as ovoid bodies that are hypointense to white matter and either isointense or diffusely hyperintense relative to CSF.[4,7,8,11,16,56] Roughly 55% to 60% of PCs appear hyperintense relative to CSF in the ventricles.[23] The hyperintensity of the cystic contents is partly attributed to the lack of flow in comparison with the surrounding CSF, remnants of previous hemorrhage, or increased protein levels within the cystic contents.[56] However, one author has noted that hyperintensity relative to CSF can be so pronounced that hemangioblastoma was considered in the differential diagnosis.[22] Although PCs do not exhibit enhancement, the surrounding remnant pineal tissue does exhibit enhancement.[10] The cyst wall appears slightly hypointense relative to the adjacent brain on T1-WI, although it is also common to appear isointense relative to adjacent structures.[40]

On contrast imaging, roughly 60% of PCs show enhancement.[15] Because of the lack of a blood-brain barrier surrounding it, the pineal tissue around the cyst can be infiltrated by gadolinium and appear hyperintense, resulting in a thin enhancement (<2 mm).[6,23] However, Fain and colleagues[17] reported an atypical nodular enhancement in their series following contrast, with Michielsen and colleagues[22] noting that the hyperintensity was more predominant posteriorly. Normally the center of the cyst does not enhance following immediate imaging after intravenous administration of contrast agent. However, gadolinium can make the PC enhance uniformly and appear solid through infiltrating and filling the avascular cyst if imaging is delayed 60 to 90 minutes, which may make differentiation between PCs and neoplastic lesions in the area difficult (see **Fig. 3**).[23,33,57] Overall, a rim enhancement pattern on MRI immediately following administration of contrast medium is suggestive of a PC rather than another pineal region lesion.[57]

On T2-WI, PCs typically have a homogeneous appearance and are isointense or slightly hyperintense relative to CSF.[4,7,8,11,16,40,56,62] Mild increases in protein content are unlikely to alter the T2-WI scans in a meaningful way, and the increased intensity is likely due to stagnant cystic contents. A cyst wall with a thickness of 2 mm or thinner[25,63] can be detected; however, some reports have found incomplete enhancement of the cyst wall that appears slightly hypointense compared with CSF on T2-WI.[6] On PD-WI, PCs typically appear slightly hyperintense or isointense to CSF.[6,21]

Although fluid-attenuated inversion recovery (FLAIR) sequences are adjusted to suppress CSF, enhancement of cystic fluids within PCs is not suppressed in the majority of cases. In an imaging study using FLAIR sequences, images of 21 out of 24 (87.5%) patients with PCs demonstrated imaging characteristics distinct from CSF. On FLAIR images, PCs do not always have signaling characteristics similar to CSF and may appear slightly hyperintense with respect to CSF.[25,63,64] In addition, signal intensity on FLAIR imaging relative to white matter is highly variable. Of 24 patients with PCs, 6 showed hypointensity, 5 showed hyperintensity, and 10 showed isointensity relative to white matter. In addition, contrast enhancement of cystic contents was not found in any patients receiving contrast (n = 18).[64]

High-Resolution MRI

Several investigators have noted the diagnostic challenges of differentiating between pineal cysts and pineal tumors.[5,20,64] Given that traditional MRI techniques commonly show the characteristic enhancing thin rim of PCs, Pastel and colleagues[64] conducted a retrospective study of PCs using high-resolution MRI to determine whether unique internal structures of PCs can be visualized and

used as a diagnostic tool. Fast imaging employing steady-state acquisition (FIESTA) sequences was used with a 1.5-T MRI unit. Sixty consecutive patients with reported PCs were reviewed at their institution, and 24 patients satisfied inclusion criteria. PCs on scans using FIESTA, available in 10 of 24 patients, typically appear hyperintense to CSF. The average age was 26 years (range 2–64 years), and the average cyst size was 13 mm across (range 8–23 mm). FIESTA studies were effective in visualizing the internal structure within the cysts. Although 4 patients showed homogeneous PCs lacking internal structure with smooth, thin walls, 6 patients showed some internal structure. One patient showed multiple small nodular cysts, 3 patients had at least one thin septation within the cyst, and 2 patients showed both multiple small cysts and internal septations. Furthermore, all PCs containing internal structures were stable during follow-up (range 5–25 months). Internal structures, such as multiple small nodular cysts and internal septations, as detected on FIESTA sequences, are common findings of PCs and are not imaging features that indicate a malignant pathology. Given the variable radiological appearance of PCs on traditional MRI, high-resolution scans capable of appreciating the internal features of PCs can aid in the differentiation between PCs and pineal tumors.[64]

Recently, Nolte and colleagues[3] conducted another retrospective imaging study to examine the diagnostic efficacy of standard and high-resolution 3-dimensional trueFISP (true fast imaging with steady-state precession) MRI sequences using a 1.5-T MRI unit. The T1-WI, T2-WI, FLAIR, and trueFISP of 111 patients randomly selected from a pool of patients undergoing MR scans were analyzed (**Fig. 4**). On trueFISP imaging, PCs are sharply defined and appear to be hypointense relative to CSF and hyperintense relative to white matter. Definite diagnoses of PCs were made more frequently with trueFISP (frequency 35.1%) compared with T1-WI (9.0%), T2-WI (4.5%), and FLAIR (9.0%), whereas the number of uncertain diagnoses was lowest in trueFISP (5.4%) compared with T1-WI (17.1%), T2-WI (11.7%), and FLAIR (16.2%). Unlike earlier imaging studies, trueFISP sequences were able to detect PCs at a rate comparable to that reported by autopsy studies (35.1% and 33%–40%, respectively).[1–3] In addition, trueFISP was found to be more sensitive for visualizing the internal structures of PCs and distinguishing atypical PCs that are defined by a rim greater than 2 mm, irregular and nonovoid shape, and/or internal trabeculations (**Fig. 5**). Of the 39 definite diagnoses of PCs detected through trueFISP, 16 (41.0%) were atypical: 6 cysts with

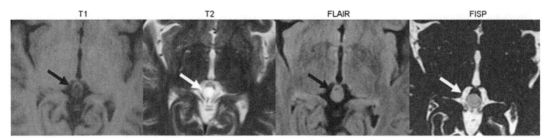

Fig. 4. Pineal cyst (*arrow*) with typical imaging features is shown on standard MR sequences and trueFISP. (*Reprinted from* Nolte I, Brockmann MA, Gerigk K, et al. TrueFISP imaging of the pineal gland: more cysts and more abnormalities. Clin Neurol Neurosurg 2010;112:205. Copyright 2010; with permission from Elsevier.)

irregular and nonovoid shape, 5 with internal trabeculations, and 5 with both of the aforementioned characteristics. However, standard sequences only detected atypical characteristics in 21.4% of PCs. High-resolution MRI using trueFISP proved to be superior to the other sequences for both detecting and visualizing the internal structures of PCs. Given the shared imaging characteristics of atypical PCs and pineal neoplasms, some investigators have suggested that atypical imaging characteristics of PCs warrant regular imaging follow-up or even surgical intervention, as atypical features appear to be common incidental findings of benign PCs.[3]

Transcranial Sonography

Transcranial sonography (TCS) is a noninvasive ultrasound-based neuroimaging technique able to generate black and white 2-dimensional planar images that depict the echogenicity of the brain parenchyma. Several studies have demonstrated the ability of TCS to visualize both the normal pineal gland and PCs.[65–67] Images are constructed to reflect variations in tissue density and depict changes in cytoarchitecture or mineral content.[65]

Harrer and colleagues[67] first demonstrated the viability of TCS as an alternative neuroimaging technique in the detection and follow-up of PCs in a case report of a patient with an asymptomatic PC incidentally detected through TCS. Imaging was performed with Sonos 5500 duplex device (Philips Medical Systems, Best, the Netherlands) and a 1.8/3.6-MHz sector transducer. B-mode ultrasound through the temporal bone window detected an ovoid PC 17 mm in diameter with an adjacent hyperechogenic region to the right. Cystic contents appeared slightly hyperechogenic relative to CSF within the third ventricle. Following administration of galactose-based contrast medium, a peak-intensity-parameter image provided an even sharper delineation of the lesion. Adjacent and surrounding healthy brain enhanced sharply whereas the cystic body of PC did not. These results corresponded with T1-WI MRI, which revealed a hypointense PC 18 mm in diameter with an atypical isointense solid nodular component that was strongly enhancing on contrast-enhanced T1-WI sequences. During 15-month follow-up, both TCS and MRI detected similar results and found no change in cyst size or appearance.

The reliability of TCS was further demonstrated in a larger study from Budisic and colleagues[65]

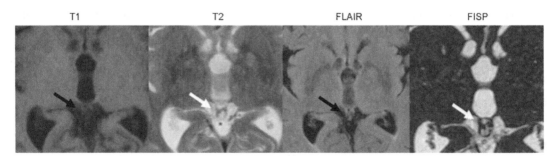

Fig. 5. Pineal cyst (*arrow*) is shown on standard MR sequences and trueFISP. Detection of a pineal cyst is clearest on T2-weighted and trueFISP imaging, and trueFISP provides superior delineation of trabeculations within the cyst. (*Reprinted from* Nolte I, Brockmann MA, Gerigk K, et al. TrueFISP imaging of the pineal gland: more cysts and more abnormalities. Clin Neurol Neurosurg 2010;112:206. Copyright 2010; with permission from Elsevier.)

of 60 patients who had received previous MRI scans. Two independent reviewers blinded to the results of the MRI scans evaluated the patients with TCS. Isonation was done through the temporal bone window using Aloka ProSound Alpha 10 (Aloka, Tokyo, Japan) and a 2-MHz sector transducer. Seven cases were excluded because of poor TCS imaging due to insufficient temporal bone windows. TCS accurately identified all cases of PCs (n = 14) and patients in the control group without pineal lesions (n = 39), as confirmed by MRI. On TCS, echogenicity of PCs is similar to CSF. PCs appear as a hypoechogenic region situated within the hyperechogenic pineal gland matrix or a hypoechogenic region bounded by a thin hyperechogenic wall. In addition, PCs may exhibit septations or peripheral hyperechogenic calcifications (**Fig. 6**). Measured differences of PC size in the pathology group were not statistically different among the two reviewers (9.55 × 7.82 vs 9.37 × 7.79 mm), nor between TCS and MRI (9.55 × 7.82 vs 9.60 × 7.67 mm). In addition, measured differences of the pineal gland size in the control groups were not statistically different between the two observers and the two imaging modalities. In a later study from the same investigators, TCS was just as effective as MRI in detecting stable disease during 2-year follow-up of PC patients.[66]

Although TCS does not appear to be able to differentiate between benign PCs and pineal tumors, the results demonstrated that TCS is comparable with MRI in the detection and follow-up of pineal cysts, especially in adults when calcification is present. Despite poorer spatial resolution than MRI and the requirement of a sufficient temporal bone window, TCS appears to be a portable, cost-effective, and reliable potential alternative to MRI particularly during follow-up for an established PC.[65,66]

SUMMARY

Differentiation between PCs and pineal tumors is not a trivial problem, particularly during earlier stages of pathology.[40] The reviewed characteristic radiological features of PCs can assist clinicians in narrowing their differential diagnosis by assessing for pineal lesions in both symptomatic and asymptomatic patients. PCs typically appear as small, well-circumscribed, unilocular masses within the pineal gland, typically measuring 5 to 15 mm in many asymptomatic patients. PCs are best visualized in a sagittal plane and either reside within or completely replace the pineal gland. PCs typically possess imaging characteristics similar to CSF, but signal intensity is variable depending on the cystic components, presence of hemorrhage, or calcification. On MRI, a thin uniform ovoid rim surrounds cystic contents that normally appear homogeneous without internal trabeculations. Mass effect is usually absent. Due to disruption of the blood-brain barrier, displaced or surrounding pineal tissue can be visualized through contrast-enhanced images, resulting in a thin enhancing rim (<2 mm). With higher-resolution imaging modalities, atypical cyst features characterized by irregular nodularity, single or multiple septations, or internal trabeculations are observed more frequently. However, these atypical internal features are common findings and are not necessarily associated malignancy or cystic growth. Although PCs are mainly found through MRI, TCS has recently been demonstrated to be a comparable imaging tool useful during follow-up imaging of PCs.

ACKNOWLEDGMENTS

Marko Spasic (third author) was partially supported by an American Association of Neurological Surgeons Fellowship grant. Isaac Yang (senior author) was partially supported by a Visionary Fund Grant and a UCLA Stein Oppenheimer grant.

REFERENCES

1. Hasegawa A, Ohtsubo K, Mori W. Pineal gland in old age; quantitative and qualitative morphological study of 168 human autopsy cases. Brain Res 1987;409(2):343–9.
2. Pu Y, Mahankali S, Hou J, et al. High prevalence of pineal cysts in healthy adults demonstrated by

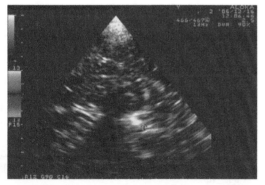

Fig. 6. Pineal cyst in a 21-year-old patient. An ovoid hypoechogenic pineal cyst (*arrow*) is seen with a sharply hyperechogenic region of calcification. (*Reprinted from* Budisic M, Bosniak J, Lovrencic-Huzjan A, et al. Pineal gland cyst evaluated by transcranial sonography. Eur J Neurol 2008;15:231. Copyright 2008; with permission from John Wiley and Sons.)

high-resolution, noncontrast brain MR imaging. AJNR Am J Neuroradiol 2007;28(9):1706–9.

3. Nolte I, Brockmann MA, Gerigk L, et al. TrueFISP imaging of the pineal gland: more cysts and more abnormalities. Clin Neurol Neurosurg 2010;112(3): 204–8.

4. Di Costanzo A, Tedeschi G, Di Salle F, et al. Pineal cysts: an incidental MRI finding? J Neurol Neurosurg Psychiatry 1993;56(2):207–8.

5. Golzarian J, Baleriaux D, Bank WO, et al. Pineal cyst: normal or pathological? Neuroradiology 1993; 35(4):251–3.

6. Jinkins JR, Xiong L, Reiter RJ. The midline pineal "eye": MR and CT characteristics of the pineal gland with and without benign cyst formation. J Pineal Res 1995;19(2):64–71.

7. Lee DH, Norman D, Newton TH. MR imaging of pineal cysts. J Comput Assist Tomogr 1987;11(4):586–90.

8. Mamourian AC, Towfighi J. Pineal cysts: MR imaging. AJNR Am J Neuroradiol 1986;7(6):1081–6.

9. Bodensteiner JB, Schaefer GB, Keller GM, et al. Incidental pineal cysts in a prospectively ascertained normal cohort. Clin Pediatr (Phila) 1996;35(5):277–9.

10. Sun B, Wang D, Tang Y, et al. The pineal volume: a three-dimensional volumetric study in healthy young adults using 3.0 T MR data. Int J Dev Neurosci 2009;27(7):655–60.

11. Sawamura Y, Ikeda J, Ozawa M, et al. Magnetic resonance images reveal a high incidence of asymptomatic pineal cysts in young women. Neurosurgery 1995;37(1):11–5 [discussion: 15-6].

12. Cooper ER. The human pineal gland and pineal cysts. J Anat 1932;67(Pt 1):28–46.

13. Hajdu SI, Porro RS, Lieberman PH, et al. Degeneration of the pineal gland of patients with cancer. Cancer 1972;29(3):706–9.

14. Megyeri L. [Cystic changes in the pineal body.] Frankf Z Pathol 1960;70:699–704 [in German].

15. Osborn AG, Preece MT. Intracranial cysts: radiologic-pathologic correlation and imaging approach. Radiology 2006;239(3):650–64.

16. Al-Holou WN, Garton HJ, Muraszko KM, et al. Prevalence of pineal cysts in children and young adults. Clinical article. J Neurosurg Pediatr 2009;4(3):230–6.

17. Fain JS, Tomlinson FH, Scheithauer BW, et al. Symptomatic glial cysts of the pineal gland. J Neurosurg 1994;80(3):454–60.

18. Klein P, Rubinstein LJ. Benign symptomatic glial cysts of the pineal gland: a report of seven cases and review of the literature. J Neurol Neurosurg Psychiatry 1989;52(8):991–5.

19. Wisoff JH, Epstein F. Surgical management of symptomatic pineal cysts. J Neurosurg 1992;77(6):896–900.

20. Fleege MA, Miller GM, Fletcher GP, et al. Benign glial cysts of the pineal gland: unusual imaging characteristics with histologic correlation. AJNR Am J Neuroradiol 1994;15(1):161–6.

21. Mena H, Armonda RA, Ribas JL, et al. Nonneoplastic pineal cysts: a clinicopathologic study of twenty-one cases. Ann Diagn Pathol 1997;1(1):11–8.

22. Michielsen G, Benoit Y, Baert E, et al. Symptomatic pineal cysts: clinical manifestations and management. Acta Neurochir (Wien) 2002;144(3):233–42 [discussion: 242].

23. Gaillard F, Jones J. Masses of the pineal region: clinical presentation and radiographic features. Postgrad Med J 2010;86(1020):597–607.

24. Barboriak DP, Lee L, Provenzale JM. Serial MR imaging of pineal cysts: implications for natural history and follow-up. AJR Am J Roentgenol 2001;176(3):737–43.

25. Tamaki N, Shirataki K, Lin TK, et al. Cysts of the pineal gland. A new clinical entity to be distinguished from tumors of the pineal region. Childs Nerv Syst 1989;5(3):172–6.

26. Kjos BO, Brant-Zawadzki M, Kucharczyk W, et al. Cystic intracranial lesions: magnetic resonance imaging. Radiology 1985;155(2):363–9.

27. Welton PL, Reicher MA, Kellerhouse LE, et al. MR of benign pineal cyst. AJNR Am J Neuroradiol 1988; 9(3):612.

28. Evans RW, Peres MF. Headaches and pineal cysts. Headache 2010;50(4):666–8.

29. Mandera M, Marcol W, Bierzynska-Macyszyn G, et al. Pineal cysts in childhood. Childs Nerv Syst 2003;19(10–11):750–5.

30. Al-Holou WN, Maher CO, Muraszko KM, et al. The natural history of pineal cysts in children and young adults. J Neurosurg Pediatr 2010;5(2):162–6.

31. Steven DA, McGinn GJ, McClarty BM. A choroid plexus papilloma arising from an incidental pineal cyst. AJNR Am J Neuroradiol 1996;17(5):939–42.

32. Hayashida Y, Hirai T, Korogi Y, et al. Pineal cystic germinoma with syncytiotrophoblastic giant cells mimicking MR imaging findings of a pineal cyst. AJNR Am J Neuroradiol 2004;25(9):1538–40.

33. Fakhran S, Escott EJ. Pineocytoma mimicking a pineal cyst on imaging: true diagnostic dilemma or a case of incomplete imaging? AJNR Am J Neuroradiol 2008;29(1):159–63.

34. Engel U, Gottschalk S, Niehaus L, et al. Cystic lesions of the pineal region—MRI and pathology. Neuroradiology 2000;42(6):399–402.

35. Seifert CL, Woeller A, Valet M, et al. Headaches and pineal cyst: a case-control study. Headache 2008; 48(3):448–52.

36. Altun A, Ugur-Altun B. Melatonin: therapeutic and clinical utilization. Int J Clin Pract 2007;61(5): 835–45.

37. Kumar KV, Verma A, Modi KD, et al. Precocious puberty and pineal cyst—an uncommon association. Indian Pediatr 2010;47(2):193–4.

38. Smirniotopoulos JG, Rushing EJ, Mena H. Pineal region masses: differential diagnosis. Radiographics 1992;12(3):577–96.

39. Peres MF, Zukerman E, Porto PP, et al. Headaches and pineal cyst: a (more than) coincidental relationship? Headache 2004;44(9):929–30.

40. Molina-Martinez FJ, Jimenez-Martinez MC, Vives-Pastor B. Some questions provoked by a chronic headache (with mixed migraine and cluster headache features) in a woman with a pineal cyst. Answers from a literature review. Cephalalgia 2010;30(9):1031–40.

41. Fetell MR, Stein BM. Neuroendocrine aspects of pineal tumors. Neurol Clin 1986;4(4):877–905.

42. Echevarria ME, Fangusaro J, Goldman S. Pediatric central nervous system germ cell tumors: a review. Oncologist 2008;13(6):690–9.

43. Masruha MR, de Souza Vieira DS, Minett TS, et al. Low urinary 6-sulphatoxymelatonin concentrations in acute migraine. J Headache Pain 2008;9(4):221–4.

44. Peres MF. Melatonin, the pineal gland and their implications for headache disorders. Cephalalgia 2005;25(6):403–11.

45. Peres MF, Masruha MR, Zukerman E, et al. Potential therapeutic use of melatonin in migraine and other headache disorders. Expert Opin Investig Drugs 2006;15(4):367–75.

46. Peres MF, Zukerman E, da Cunha Tanuri F, et al. Melatonin, 3 mg, is effective for migraine prevention. Neurology 2004;63(4):757.

47. Tanuri FC, de Lima E, Peres MF, et al. Melatonin treatment decreases c-fos expression in a headache model induced by capsaicin. J Headache Pain 2009;10(2):105–10.

48. Leone M, D'Amico D, Moschiano F, et al. Melatonin versus placebo in the prophylaxis of cluster headache: a double-blind pilot study with parallel groups. Cephalalgia 1996;16(7):494–6.

49. Tapp E. The histology and pathology of the human pineal gland. Prog Brain Res 1979;52:481–500.

50. Tajima Y, Minami N, Sudo K, et al. Hot water epilepsy with pineal cyst and cavum septi pellucidi. Jpn J Psychiatry Neurol 1993;47(1):111–4.

51. Milroy CM, Smith CL. Sudden death due to a glial cyst of the pineal gland. J Clin Pathol 1996;49(3):267–9.

52. Richardson JK, Hirsch CS. Sudden, unexpected death due to "pineal apoplexy". Am J Forensic Med Pathol 1986;7(1):64–8.

53. Morgan JT, Scumpia AJ, Webster TM, et al. Resting tremor secondary to a pineal cyst: case report and review of the literature. Pediatr Neurosurg 2008; 44(3):234–8.

54. Kitayama J, Toyoda K, Fujii K, et al. Recurrent aseptic meningitis caused by rupture of a pineal cyst. No To Shinkei 1996;48(12):1147–50 [in Japanese].

55. Di Chirico A, Di Rocco F, Velardi F. Spontaneous regression of a symptomatic pineal cyst after endoscopic third-ventriculostomy. Childs Nerv Syst 2001; 17(1–2):42–6.

56. Korogi Y, Takahashi M, Ushio Y. MRI of pineal region tumors. J Neurooncol 2001;54(3):251–61.

57. Sener RN. The pineal gland: a comparative MR imaging study in children and adults with respect to normal anatomical variations and pineal cysts. Pediatr Radiol 1995;25(4):245–8.

58. Musolino A, Cambria S, Rizzo G, et al. Symptomatic cysts of the pineal gland: stereotactic diagnosis and treatment of two cases and review of the literature. Neurosurgery 1993;32(2):315–20 [discussion: 320–1].

59. Todo T, Kondo T, Shinoura N, et al. Large cysts of the pineal gland: report of two cases. Neurosurgery 1991;29(1):101–5 [discussion: 105–6].

60. Tapp E, Huxley M. The histological appearance of the human pineal gland from puberty to old age. J Pathol 1972;108(2):137–44.

61. Mamourian AC, Yarnell T. Enhancement of pineal cysts on MR images. AJNR Am J Neuroradiol 1991;12(4):773–4.

62. Sandhu JS, McLaughlin JR, Gomez CR. Characteristics of incidental pineal cysts on magnetic resonance imaging. Neurosurgery 1989;25(4):636–9 [discussion: 640].

63. Bosnjak J, Budisic M, Azman D, et al. Pineal gland cysts—an overview. Acta Clin Croat 2009;48(3):355–8.

64. Pastel DA, Mamourian AC, Duhaime AC. Internal structure in pineal cysts on high-resolution magnetic resonance imaging: not a sign of malignancy. J Neurosurg Pediatr 2009;4(1):81–4.

65. Budisic M, Bosnjak J, Lovrencic-Huzjan A, et al. Pineal gland cyst evaluated by transcranial sonography. Eur J Neurol 2008;15(3):229–33.

66. Budisic M, Bosnjak J, Lovrencic-Huzjan A, et al. Transcranial sonography in the evaluation of pineal lesions: two-year follow up study. Acta Clin Croat 2008;47(4):205–10.

67. Harrer JU, Klotzsch C, Oertel MF, et al. Sonographic detection and follow up of an atypical pineal cyst: a comparison with magnetic resonance imaging [case report]. J Neurosurg 2005;103(3):564–6.

Preoperative Evaluation of Pineal Tumors

Jonathon J. Parker, BS, Allen Waziri, MD*

KEYWORDS

- Pineal region • Pineal gland • Pineal tumors
- Preoperative evaluation

The pineal gland, a small pinecone-shaped structure, named *konareion* by the Greek physician Galen, is a unique organ whose diverse functions are not completely understood.[1] The gland measures on average $7 \times 6 \times 3$ mm and is composed predominantly of pineocytes (retinal photoreceptor-like cells), which are divided by highly vascular septa.[2] The gland does not retain the normal blood brain barrier, allowing it to enhance with contrast material on CT and MRI.[3] The pineal gland is presumed to function in transduction of neural inputs relayed from the retina via the suprachiasmatic nucleus and superior cervical ganglion into coordinated melatonin secretion from the pineocytes, thereby regulating the diurnal sleep-wake cycle.[1] The pineal glad and surrounding structures of the pineal region are primarily of interest to neurosurgeons due to the incidence of a variety of neoplastic lesions that occur in this area.

This review focuses on several critical aspects of the preoperative evaluation of pineal masses: radiographic diagnostics, considerations in preoperative strategic planning, and tumor marker tests and their interpretation. These concepts are critical not only for maximizing diagnostic and prognostic information for patients with pineal region tumors but also in optimizing operative safety and in the initiation of appropriate oncologic consultation and management.

CLINICAL PRESENTATION AND SYMPTOMATOLOGY

Pineal tumors constitute 1% of all central nervous system tumors in adults and 3% to 8% of central nervous system tumors in children.[4,5] Masses in the pineal region can present with headaches, nausea, and vomiting consistent with increased intracranial pressure due to obstructive hydrocephalus from compression of the cerebral aqueduct. On average, patients exhibit symptoms 11 months before diagnosis with a pineal region mass.[6] These patients often require cerebrospinal fluid (CSF) shunting or ostomy of the floor of the third ventricle to resolve obstructive hydrocephalus. Pineal region tumors can also induce cerebellar and midbrain signs due to either mass effect or direct brain invasion. Pineal masses located at the dorsal midbrain often compress the tectal plate, resulting in Parinaud syndrome. In the largest case series to date, of 700 patients with pineal region tumors, the most common clinical presentation was increased intracranial pressure (87% of the cases), followed by eye movement disorders (76%), and lastly cerebellar signs (52%).[6] On rare occasions pineal masses present with sleep-wake cycle disturbances and psychosis.[7,8]

PREOPERATIVE RADIOGRAPHIC IMAGING FOR PATIENTS WITH PINEAL TUMORS

In the modern age, pineal region masses are easily identified on cranial imaging. The differential diagnosis for radiographic abnormalities found within the pineal region can be divided into 3 categories: benign cysts, tumors of the pineal region, and rare pathologies.[5] When a pineal region mass is suspected or identified on cranial imaging, the gold standard for thorough preoperative imaging evaluation is full craniospinal MRI with intravenous

Disclosures: None.
Department of Neurosurgery, University of Colorado School of Medicine, Academic Office Building, Room 5001, 12631 East, 17th Avenue, Aurora, CO 80045, USA
* Corresponding author.
E-mail address: allen.waziri@ucdenver.edu

Neurosurg Clin N Am 22 (2011) 353–358
doi:10.1016/j.nec.2011.04.003
1042-3680/11/$ – see front matter © 2011 Elsevier Inc. All rights reserved.

contrast administration. Preoperative imaging of the spinal column is critical, given the proclivity of malignant lesions to seed metastases within the spinal canal and perturbation of postoperative imaging studies after an intradural neurosurgical procedure. This article focuses on radiographic characteristics of pineal region masses associated with prognostic data and preoperative surgical planning.

Imaging Characteristics of Normal and Pathologic Entities of the Pineal Gland

Normal pineal gland

The normal pineal gland is often easy to visualize on CT imaging due to calcification and the resulting hyperdensity. The percentage of patients with calcification increases with age and peaks between 20 and 40 years of age when 33% to 40% of patients have a calcified gland.[9] Pineal calcification alone does not differentiate between a normal and pathologic gland.

Pineal cysts

Pineal cysts are a benign entity, are 3 times more common in female patients, and can be seen on 1.4% to 10% of all cranial MRIs.[10] The majority of these cysts are less than 10 mm in size, asymptomatic, and remain stable in size over time.[11] Larger cysts are commonly seen, however, and more likely to approach clinical presentation due to localized mass effect. On CT scanning, these lesions tend to be hypodense, with occasional (25%) rim calcification.[10] On T1 MRI, half are hypointense and half hyperintense to CSF, making T2 signal hyperintensity and partial signal attenuation on fluid-attenuated inversion recovery of more diagnostic use.[5,10] Up to 60% of pineal cysts demonstrate peripherally located gadolinium contrast enhancement. Pineal cysts can be difficult to differentiate from pineal region tumors, given their proximity to the internal cerebral veins, making the interpretation of mass versus vascular enhancement challenging.[9] There has been debate in the literature as to whether asymptomatic pineal cysts can be followed clinically or require serial imaging[9,11]; however, the majority of surgeons in the modern age do not recommend serial imaging for patients with simple and otherwise asymptomatic pineal cysts.

Germ cell tumors

Germ cell tumors are the most common pineal region tumor and account for 31% to 85% of all pineal tumors.[4,6] These tumors fall into germinomatous and nongerminomatous categories, with a higher incidence of germinomatous tumors. Germinomas arise from entrapped totipotent germ cells. In 90% of cases, these tumors present in patients under 20 years of age.[5] These tumors have a marked male to female predominance, ranging from 5:1 to 22:1.[3,5] CSF dissemination occurs commonly and requires full craniospinal MRI to evaluate for the presence of drop metastases. On CT imaging, these tumors are generally hyperdense with sharp borders and seem to engulf the pineal gland and the associated intrinsic calcifications. In 43% of cases, the pathognmonic butterfly sign can be visualized on both CT and MRI, as the tumor infiltrates laterally with subependymal infiltration of the thalamus.[6] On T1-weighted and T2-weighted MRI, these tumors tend to be isointense to gray matter, although there are exceptions.[9] These masses can be cystic and are commonly contrast enhancing.[12] Synchronous germinomas within the pituitary or suprasellar region have also been described, which may potentially result in pituitary dysfunction and mandate a thorough preoperative hormonal evaluation in affected patients.[13,14]

Nongerminomatous germ cell tumors encompass the less common totipotent germ cell malignancies, including teratoma, choriocarcinoma, yolk sac tumors, embryonal carcinoma, and mixed germ cell tumors. These tumors, as a category, harbor worse prognoses than pure germinoma, with durable tumor remission in only 66% of patients.[5] The bad actors of this group include choriocarcinoma, embryonal carcinoma, and yolk sac tumors, all of which portend a meager 3-year survival rate of only 27%.[15] Imaging presentation of these masses is variable, but they are generally isodense or hyperdense to gray matter.[16] Of radiographic interest, choriocarcinomas have a proclivity for hemorrhage (resulting in the presence of hypointense components on gradient-echo sequences) and teratomas demonstrate a high incidence of calcification.

Pineal parenchymal tumors

Pineal parenchymal tumors (PPTs) account for 15% of all pineal tumors and arise directly from pineocytes. PPTs have been classically divided into 2 entities, pineocytomas and pineoblastomas.[5] As of 2007, however, the World Health Organization criteria now recognize 3 PPT entities, including pineocytoma (I), PPT of intermediate differentiation (II and III), and pineoblastoma (IV). Pineocytomas are a grade I lesion, predominantly identified in adults (mean onset at 38 years of age), and grow in a slow and circumscribed manner, making them amenable to cure by gross total resection.[3] Pineoblastomas make up 40% of all PPTs and are most common in the pediatric population, with a mean age of presentation of 12.6 years.[17] As the most malignant PPT with the worst prognosis, pineoblastoma frequently disseminates through the CSF and has a reported 5-year survival rate of 58% to 62%.[9,18] CSF dissemination of pineoblastoma has been reported in 14% to 43% of cases,[19] again mandating the need for full preoperative MRI of the entire neuroaxis. PPTs of intermediate differentiation reside along the pathologic continuum between pineocytoma and pineoblastoma, have intermediate prognosis and pathologic features, and comprise 20% of all PPTs.[3]

On noncontrast CT imaging, pineoblastomas and pineocytomas tend to appear hyperdense due to their relative hypercellularity compared with surrounding tissue. The canonical pattern of exploded calcification is thought to result from tumor mass pressing intrinsic pineal calcifications to more superficial locations, in contrast to the engulfed appearance of germinoma calcification.[5] The high-grade pineoblastoma, in contrast to the lower-grade pineocytoma, is more likely to be larger, have indications of hemorrhage, and demonstrate irregular borders with brain invasion.[9] It is difficult to differentiate between the pineoblastoma and pineocytoma on imaging alone, although the pineocytoma is more often smaller and calcified.[9] On MRI, there is considerable variation in the appearance of these lesions, although pineoblastoma tends to be isointense to gray matter on T2 and pineocytoma has a comparatively higher intensity.[20] PPTs of intermediate differentiation have no unique imaging characteristics. It is important to recognize that there are no pathognomonic imaging characteristics or reliable serum of CSF tests for PPTs, thus mandating tissue biopsy for definitive diagnosis.

Papillary tumor of the pineal region
The papillary tumor of the pineal region is a newly recognized pathologic entity thought to arise from ependymocytes of the subcomissural organ.[21] This neoplasm has yet to be assigned a World Health Organization grade but has a median age of presentation of 29 and a 5-year survival of 73%.[3,22,23] These lesions have varying T1 intensity and marked T2 hyperintensity, with cystic areas common. These tumors tend to recur locally despite surgical resection and rarely exhibit CSF dissemination (7%).[3]

Glioma
Although not as common as germ cell tumors, gliomas often occur in the pineal region and arise from surrounding brain structures, including the tectal plate (eg, tectal gliomas), the midbrain, and the cerebellum rather than from the resident stromal astrocytes of the pineal gland.[20] Tectal gliomas are prevalent in the pediatric population, are commonly low grade, progress slowly, and are frequently managed by shunting and observation alone. These exophytic lesions can enhance on postcontrast CT and MRI but this does not indicate the grade of the neoplasm.[4] Other glial lineage neoplasms occur in the pineal region, including ependymomas.

Rare pathologies
A comprehensive review of all pineal masses is outside the scope of this review. The pineal region harbors a range of more rare pathologies, including meningioma, hemangiopericytoma, lipoma, metastasis, infection, venous aneurysm, vascular malformation, sarcoidosis, and others. Each of these entities has unique clinical and neuroradiologic presentations.[5,21,24]

SURGICAL CONSIDERATIONS DERIVED FROM PREOPERATIVE IMAGING

There are 2 major presurgical implications when considering cranial imaging for patients with pineal region masses. The first that must be considered in presurgical evaluation is the presence of obstructive hydrocephalus due to compression of the aqueduct or posterior aspect of the third ventricle. Patients with pineal masses may present with symptoms of hydrocephalus that may be relatively acute in nature; in contrast, patients with more chronic compression may demonstrate evidence of profound ventriculomegaly in the setting of relatively benign symptomatology. In the latter case, it may be presumed that the pineal region mass may be more slow growing in nature and that the potential for rapid clinical deterioration due to hydrocephalus may be somewhat less likely. In either case, the presence of hydrocephalus on preoperative imaging warrants consideration of either temporary or permanent CSF diversion. Management of hydrocephalus for patients with pineal tumors depends to a great extent on the experience and personal preference of the operating neurosurgeon. In cases of predicted significant resection of the pineal mass, many surgeons place a temporary external ventricular drain (EVD) at the initiation of the planned definitive resection. In this case, CSF can be obtained before resection for the purposes of diagnostic analyses (discussed later). Alternatively, many surgeons (particularly in the pediatric world) advocate for endoscopic third ventriculostomy before surgery on pineal region masses that cause obstructive hydrocephalus. CSF for diagnostic studies can be similarly obtained in preoperative fashion during ventricular access for these procedures. Finally, in cases of anatomic characteristics of the prepontine cistern or other structures precluding endoscopic third ventriculostomy, definitive ventriculoperitoneal shunting may be used.

The second preoperative consideration that can be derived from evaluation of cranial MRI is the decision regarding surgical approach. In the setting of imaging and diagnostic criteria that are supportive of germinoma, simple stereotactic biopsy of the lesion is the appropriate surgical decision. In the majority of cases, however, an open surgical approach is warranted. Several elements of the local anatomy are critical for review when evaluating the surgical approach, including the angle of the tentorium and the relationship of the deep venous system to the tumor. Detailed discussion of these factors is outside the scope of this review and further outlined in articles within this publication focusing on surgical approaches to the pineal region.

INTERPRETATION OF SERUM AND CSF DIAGNOSTIC TESTS FOR PINEAL REGION MASSES

Other than pituitary tumors, there is no other category of intracranial tumor for which preoperative evaluation of laboratory tests is more critical and of significant clinical utility. Preoperative work-up of patients with suspected germ cell tumors should include laboratory testing for serum and CSF levels of relevant oncoproteins, including the β subunit of human chorionic gonadotropin (β-hCG), α-fetoprotein (AFP), and (where possible) placental alkaline phosphatase (PLAP). It is preferable that testing be performed on samples obtained on the same day.[25] The biologic rationale for these tests is derived from the ability of germ cell tumors to reactivate their developmental secretion state. Thus, the yolk sac endoderm secretes AFP; syncytiotrophoblast cells secrete the glycoprotein hormone β-hCG; and syncytiotrophoblast and primitive germ cells secrete PLAP.[26] PLAP levels can be diagnostically useful, because this marker is uniquely found within CSF samples from patients with pure germinoma; unfortunately, testing for PLAP is not yet widely available.[25,27] In addition to diagnostic utility, measurement of preoperative oncoprotein levels serves as a critical baseline for subsequent tracking of the effectiveness of surgery, radiation, and chemotherapy and to monitor for tumor recurrence.[6] **Table 1** summarizes common oncoprotein trends in both the CSF and serum of germ cell tumor patients.

There is no widely accepted uniform diagnostic level for CSF and serum oncoproteins in specific germ cell tumor subtypes. CSF levels at

Table 1
CSF and serum oncoprotein markers in pineal germ cell tumors[a]

Tumor	β-hCG	AFP	PLAP
Pure Germinoma	+ (CSF)	−	+ (CSF)
Choriocarcinoma	+	−	±
Yolk Sac tumor	±	±	−
Embryonal carcinoma	Variable		
Mature teratoma	−	−	−
Immature Teratoma	±	±	−
Mixed GCT	Variable		

[a] For pure germinoma, β-hCG and PLAP are usually only detectable in the CSF when present.
Data from Refs.[3,4,15,25]

presentation are generally higher than serum levels, and elevation in CSF oncoprotein levels occurs earlier than similar elevations in serum in the setting of treatment failure.[25] Normal levels are generally thought to be less than 1.5 IU/L or 1 IU/L for β-hCG, however, and less than 1.5 ng/mL for AFP.[28] These values should be used as a guide, because there are minor variations between reference laboratories due to assay-dependent variations. Some groups have adopted a classification system using good, intermediate, and poor prognosis categories based on levels of oncoproteins in the serum and CSF.[28,29] Other groups, however, have adopted a secreting and nonsecreting GCT classification. Lastly, it has been shown that increasing amounts of either AFP and β-hCG, especially in cases where levels reach 10-fold over normal, correlate with a worse patient prognosis and increased chance of craniospinal dissemination.[30] **Table 2** summarizes the relevant laboratory value ranges and subsequent classifications.

In addition to assessment of tumor marker levels, it is recommended that CSF cytologic analysis is performed to assess for CSF tumor spread, particularly when there is clinical suspicion of a more malignant pathology, in cases of abnormal spinal neuroimaging findings, or in the presence of elevated oncoprotein levels.[25] From a research standpoint, there has been recent interest in using levels of soluble c-Kit receptor within the CSF as a marker for germinoma, primarily derived from data demonstrating high levels of this marker in patients with subarachnoid spread.[26,31] There are currently no accepted CSF or serum markers with sensitivity and specificity for PPTs, making tissue diagnosis mandatory when these tumors are suspected.

Several critical caveats must be considered in the review of oncoprotein levels from patients

Table 2
Serum and CSF oncoprotein levels for germ cell tumors and their classifications

	AFP	β-hCG
Good Prognosis	<20 ng/mL	<1.0 mIU/mL
Intermediate Prognosis	20–2000 ng/mL	>1.0 mIU/mL
Poor Prognosis	>2000 ng/mL	>2000 mIU/mL
Nonsecreting	<50 IU/L (CSF) Undetectable (serum)	<50 IU/L (CSF) Undetectable (serum)
Secreting	>50 IU/L (CSF) Any (serum)	>50 IU/L (CSF) Any (serum)

Data from Balmaceda C, Finlay J. Current advances in the diagnosis and management of intracranial germ cell tumors. Curr Neurol Neurosci Rep 2004;4(3):253–62; and Kanamori M, Kumabe T, Tominaga T. Is histologic diagnosis necessary to start treatment for germ cell tumours in the pineal region? J Clin Neurosci 2008;15(9):978–87.

with pineal region masses. First, postresection testing of serum and CSF markers is generally considered to provide significantly decreased diagnostic relevance, strongly emphasizing the need for careful preoperative imaging review and acquisition of appropriate test samples. Second, CSF levels of the various oncoproteins are generally considered more diagnostically sensitive than levels in corresponding serum samples. In cases of severe obstructive hydrocephalus, CSF testing may be deferred until ventricular access is obtained during EVD placement or EVD at the time of surgery. Most neurosurgeons, however, are comfortable with a small-volume diagnostic lumbar puncture in the majority of cases. Finally, although measurement of oncoproteins in serum and CSF may be diagnostically suggestive, the considerable variability in the pattern of marker secretion prohibits definitive diagnosis and mandates tissue biopsy for final confirmation.

SUMMARY

The role of the neurosurgeon is critical for initiating careful and responsible preoperative evaluation and care for patients with pineal region tumors. The preoperative evaluation of pineal region tumor can be simplified into a checklist: (1) evaluation for emergent surgical intervention due to symptomatic obstructive hydrocephalus or mass effect; (2) development of a focused differential after acquisition of craniospinal MRI, serum and CSF oncoprotein levels, and CSF cytology; and (3) decision on whether a biopsy, surgical resection, or both are

necessary. Subsequent biopsy or surgical resection is generally the critical first step of tumor management and leads to coordination of appropriate consultation with medical and radiation oncology.

REFERENCES

1. Macchi MM, Bruce JN. Human pineal physiology and functional significance of melatonin. Front Neuroendocrinol 2004;25(3–4):177–95.
2. Sumida M, Barkovich AJ, Newton TH. Development of the pineal gland: measurement with MR. AJNR Am J Neuroradiol 1996;17(2):233–6.
3. Smith AB, Rushing EJ, Smirniotopoulos JG. From the archives of the AFIP: lesions of the pineal region: radiologic-pathologic correlation. Radiographics 2010;30(7):2001–20.
4. Blakeley JO, Grossman SA. Management of pineal region tumors. Curr Treat Options Oncol 2006;7(6): 505–16.
5. Gaillard F, Jones J. Masses of the pineal region: clinical presentation and radiographic features. Postgrad Med J 2010;86(1020):597–607.
6. Konovalov AN, Pitskhelauri DI. Principles of treatment of the pineal region tumors. Surg Neurol 2003;59(4):250–68.
7. Mittal VA, Karlsgodt K, Zinberg J, et al. Identification and treatment of a pineal region tumor in an adolescent with prodromal psychotic symptoms. Am J Psychiatry 2010;167(9):1033–7.
8. Quera-Salva MA, Hartley S, Claustrat B, et al. Circadian rhythm disturbances associated with psychiatric symptoms in a patient with a pineal region tumor. Am J Psychiatry 2011;168(1):99–100.
9. Yousem DM, Grossman RI. Neuroradiology: the requisites. 3rd edition. Philadelphia: Mosby/Elsevier; 2010.
10. Osborn AG, Preece MT. Intracranial cysts: radiologic-pathologic correlation and imaging approach. Radiology 2006;239(3):650–64.
11. Barboriak DP, Lee L, Provenzale JM. Serial MR imaging of pineal cysts: implications for natural history and follow-up. AJR Am J Roentgenol 2001; 176(3):737–43.
12. Smirniotopoulos JG, Rushing EJ, Mena H. Pineal region masses: differential diagnosis. Radiographics 1992;12(3):577–96.
13. Cunliffe CH, Fischer I, Karajannis M, et al. Synchronous mixed germ cell tumor of the pineal gland and suprasellar region with a predominant angiomatous component: a diagnostic challenge. J Neurooncol 2009;93(2):269–74.
14. Lee L, Saran F, Hargrave D, et al. Germinoma with synchronous lesions in the pineal and suprasellar regions. Childs Nerv Syst 2006;22(12):1513–8.
15. Kyritsis AP. Management of primary intracranial germ cell tumors. J Neurooncol 2010;96(2):143–9.

16. Louis DN, Deutsches Krebsforschungszentrum Heidelberg, ebrary Inc, et al. WHO classification of tumours of the central nervous system. World Health Organization classification of tumours. 4th edition. Geneva (Switzerland): Distributed by WHO Press, World Health Organization; 2007. Available at: http://site.ebrary.com/lib/yale/Doc?id=10214529. Accessed February 20, 2011.

17. Mena H, Rushing EJ, Ribas JL, et al. Tumors of pineal parenchymal cells: a correlation of histological features, including nucleolar organizer regions, with survival in 35 cases. Hum Pathol 1995;26(1):20–30.

18. Lutterbach J, Fauchon F, Schild SE, et al. Malignant pineal parenchymal tumors in adult patients: patterns of care and prognostic factors. Neurosurgery 2002;51(1):44–55 [discussion: 55–6].

19. Grossman RI, Yousem DM. Neuroradiology: the requisites. St Louis (MO): Mosby; 1994.

20. Korogi Y, Takahashi M, Ushio Y. MRI of pineal region tumors. J Neurooncol 2001;54(3):251–61.

21. Dahiya S, Perry A. Pineal tumors. Adv Anat Pathol 2010;17(6):419–27.

22. Fevre-Montange M, Hasselblatt M, Figarella-Branger D, et al. Prognosis and histopathologic features in papillary tumors of the pineal region: a retrospective multicenter study of 31 cases. J Neuropathol Exp Neurol 2006;65(10):1004–11.

23. Lechapt-Zalcman E, Chapon F, Guillamo JS, et al. Long-term clinicopathological observations on a papillary tumour of the pineal region. Neuropathol Appl Neurobiol 2010. [Epub ahead of print].

24. Spallone A, Pitskhelauri DI. Lipomas of the pineal region. Surg Neurol 2004;62(1):52–8 [discussion: 58–9].

25. Balmaceda C, Finlay J. Current advances in the diagnosis and management of intracranial germ cell tumors. Curr Neurol Neurosci Rep 2004;4(3): 253–62.

26. Takeshima H, Kuratsu J. A review of soluble c-kit (s-kit) as a novel tumor marker and possible molecular target for the treatment of CNS germinoma. Surg Neurol 2003;60(4):321–4 [discussion: 324–5].

27. Ramakrishnan S, Manifold IH, Ward AM, et al. CSF placental alkaline phosphatase as marker in cranial dysgerminoma. Lancet 1989;2(8656):225.

28. Kanamori M, Kumabe T, Tominaga T. Is histological diagnosis necessary to start treatment for germ cell tumours in the pineal region? J Clin Neurosci 2008;15(9):978–87.

29. Kamoshima Y, Sawamura Y. Update on current standard treatments in central nervous system germ cell tumors. Curr Opin Neurol 2010;23(6):571–5.

30. Nishizaki T, Kajiwara K, Adachi N, et al. Detection of craniospinal dissemination of intracranial germ cell tumours based on serum and cerebrospinal fluid levels of tumour markers. J Clin Neurosci 2001; 8(1):27–30.

31. Miyanohara O, Takeshima H, Kaji M, et al. Diagnostic significance of soluble c-kit in the cerebrospinal fluid of patients with germ cell tumors. J Neurosurg 2002;97(1):177–83.

Stereotactic Biopsy Considerations for Pineal Tumors

Brad E. Zacharia, MD[a,*], Jeffrey N. Bruce, MD[b]

KEYWORDS

• Pineal tumors • Biopsy • Stereotactic • Pineal region

Pineal region tumors are rare, accounting for 0.4% to 1.0% of intracranial tumors in American and European literature and 4% in Japanese literature.[1,2] A myriad of tumor subtypes arise in this region, which reflects the heterogeneous nature of the pineal gland.[3–7] The pineal region lies deep within the cranium, and is closely related to the brainstem and the critical deep venous structures, and the complexities of which have led to a long-standing debate regarding the management of both benign and malignant lesions in this location.[7] Except in rare instances of elevated germ cell markers where histologic confirmation is not necessary, a rational management strategy for pineal region lesions almost always begins by obtaining a tissue diagnosis. A histologic diagnosis can be obtained via direct operative approaches, stereotactic biopsy, and endoscopic transventricular approaches, with the primary objective being establishment of an accurate histologic diagnosis.[8] Given the wide variety of histologic subtypes and mixed tumor pathologies, diagnostic accuracy is essential for making enlightened management decisions. In addition to important prognostic significance, the histologic subtype drives the use of adjuvant therapy, need for metastatic workup, and follow-up decisions. This review focuses specifically on the indications, methodology, accuracy, and safety of stereotactic biopsy for pineal region lesions.

PRINCIPLES OF STEREOTACTIC BIOPSY

Background

Frame-based stereotactic systems translate a point on a 2-dimensional image into a 3-dimensional target. There are many frame-based stereotactic systems, with the Cosman-Roberts-Wells (CRW) (Integra Lifesciences Corp, Plainsboro, NJ, USA) frame among the most popular. The CRW works on an arc radius system, allowing the aiming arc to be moved in 3 spatial places according to the obtained target coordinates. Thus, the focal point of the arc corresponds with the target. Other popular frames include the Leksell (Elekta, Stockholm) and the Brown-Roberts-Wells (BRW).[9]

Patient Selection

Unless CSF or serum markers are positive, thereby confirming a diagnosis of a malignant germ cell tumor, surgical intervention in all patients with pineal region lesions is advocated. The initial surgical decision frequently involves choosing between stereotactic biopsy and open microsurgical procedures. Zealous advocates can be found for either strategy; however, each modality is most effective when used for specific indications rather than applied exclusively for all lesions. Open resection facilitates the maximal removal of tumor volume and provides the benefits of diagnostic accuracy and, in many cases, improved

The authors have nothing to disclose.

[a] Department of Neurological Surgery, Columbia University, 710 West 168th Street, 4th Floor, New York, NY 10032, USA

[b] Department of Neurological Surgery, Columbia University College of Physicians and Surgeons, Room 434, Neurological Institute, Columbia University Medical Center, 710 West 168th Street, New York, NY 10032, USA

* Corresponding author.

E-mail address: bez2103@columbia.edu

Neurosurg Clin N Am 22 (2011) 359–366

doi:10.1016/j.nec.2011.05.008

1042-3680/11/$ – see front matter © 2011 Elsevier Inc. All rights reserved.

prognosis.[7,8] Stereotactic biopsy has the advantage of being less invasive, can be performed without the need for general anesthesia, and is associated with an overall lower risk of complications. Stereotactic biopsy is, therefore, favored in patients whose medical comorbidities preclude open surgical resection, patients with multiple lesions, and in the setting of lesions with radiographic evidence of brainstem invasion where open surgery may be of limited value.[8] Further indications include a presentation suggestive of an infectious etiology or of metastatic cancer associated with diffuse systemic disease.[10] Although most pineal region lesions may be safely biopsied, an individual analysis must be made based on the lesion's location, size, and composition, paying close attention to adjacent neural and vascular structures.

Biopsy Technique

The safety of transit through the brain has been greatly improved by modern imaging and planning software that facilitates the preoperative reconstruction of the stereotactic trajectory. Many variations and nuances exist in the actual performance of stereotactic biopsies of deep-seated lesions at various institutions; however, the basic principles are consistent. As part of their initial evaluation, patients undergo fine-cut contrast-enhanced magnetic resonance imaging (MRI) of the brain. This MRI allows for an in-depth analysis of the lesion in question, and including a fine-cut sequence provides the substrate for accurate image reconstruction during stereotactic planning. On the day of the surgery, a CRW frame is placed (typically with local anesthesia and no sedation) in the preoperative area. After obtaining a fine-cut computed tomography (CT) or MRI scan, patients are transported to the operating room. Alternatively, the frame may be placed with the aid of monitored anesthesia care or under general anesthesia, if necessary, and then transported to radiology for imaging with anesthesia. Patients are then positioned on the operating room table in the supine position with the head neutral, slightly elevated, and fixed to a Mayfield adapter to ensure rigid fixation during the biopsy procedure.

Concurrently, the stereotactic planning is performed on a computer workstation located within the operating room sterile core. The authors' institution currently uses Brainlab iPlan Stereotaxy (Brainlab, Westchester, IL, USA) for stereotactic planning, but several commercially available platforms are available. First, the CRW frame is localized within the computer system. Then the CT and MRI scans are merged using commercially available software. Although auto-merge features are used, the accuracy of the merge must be confirmed by the surgeon to ensure an accurate and safe plan before proceeding with the target/trajectory selection.

The pineal region is roughly defined as the area of the brain bounded by the splenium of the corpus callosum and the tela choroidea dorsally, the quadrigeminal plate and tectum of the midbrain ventrally, the posterior aspect of the third ventricle rostrally, and the vermis of the cerebellum caudally.[11] Targets are generally selected within regions of avid contrast enhancement, preferably in the center of the lesion to facilitate placement of the midpoint of the window of a Nashold biopsy needle (Integra Lifesciences Corp, Plainsboro, NJ, USA) within the lesion. Various trajectories can be used based on preoperative imaging, which, in the current era, would include a contrast-enhanced MRI study, although the majority of older studies relied on CT imaging. The biopsy trajectory can be orthogonal lateral, oblique anterolateral (anterolateral superior), or posterolateral (**Fig. 1**). Although no data convincingly demonstrate the superiority of one trajectory over another, a low frontal approach that stays below the internal cerebral veins is ideal and is the most commonly used approach.[11,12] This trajectory traverses the frontal lobe and internal capsule such that optimal entry points and targets can be chosen to minimize pathways through ependymal surfaces and adjacent vasculature.[8,10] A posterolateral approach via the parieto-occipital junction can be used, but is probably most appropriate for lesions with significant lateral and superior extension.

After the target and entry points are chosen, a probe's-eye view is used to ensure that pial, ependymal, and vascular elements are avoided and that the frame is set according to the determined coordinates. In the operating room, all frame settings and measurements must be meticulously checked. The use of a phantom system with the CRW frame is particularly helpful to ensure that all instruments are confirmed with reference to the target point. Once patients are properly sedated, the procedure may proceed. The importance of skillful neuroanesthesia cannot be overstated to allow for a safe biopsy.[9] Local anesthesia with mild sedation is usually sufficient and further minimizes morbidity associated with general anesthesia while allowing for periodic neurologic assessment of patients. Access to the cranium can be obtained via a twist drill or through a more substantial burr hole at the proposed entry site. A small burr hole is favored to allow for direct visualization to avoid possible entry through a sulcus; however, either approach is reasonable.

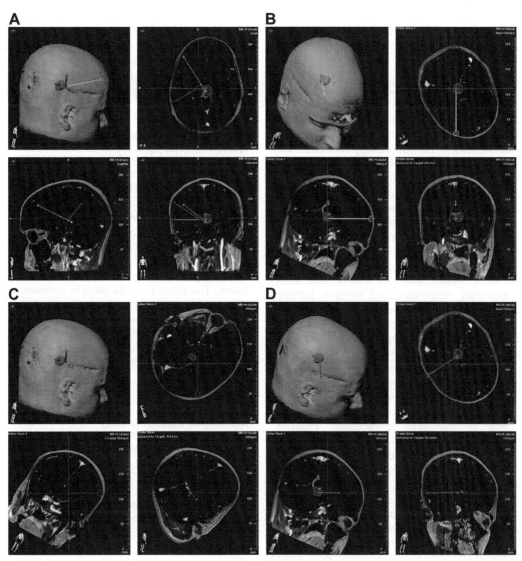

Fig. 1. Stereotactic trajectory plans using Brainlab iPlan Stereotaxy software. (*A*) Trajectory overview (*anterolateral is green, orthogonal lateral is orange, parieto-occipital is pink, and pineal lesion outlined in pink*), clockwise beginning from the upper-left panel, the authors demonstrate a 3-dimensional reconstruction, axial, coronal, and sagittal images; (*B–D* clockwise beginning from the upper-left panel, the authors demonstrate a 3-dimensional reconstruction, in-line view, probe's-eye view, and an alternative in-line view); (*B*) anterolateral or low-anterior trajectory is used for the majority of pineal region lesions and was the trajectory used in this particular case; (*C*) parieto-occipital trajectory can be used with lesions that extend laterally and superiorly, and would not be ideal for the lesion shown in these images; (*D*) orthogonal lateral trajectory is less ideal, requiring traversing temporalis muscle, and is technically more difficult using a stereotactic frame.

A Nashold side-cutting biopsy needle is used to obtain the specimen. After passing the biopsy needle to the proper depth, a small amount of suction is applied and held for several seconds before the rotation of the inner sleeve to amputate the specimen. The specimen is evacuated using a gentle saline irrigation through the biopsy needle. To begin, 2 samples are routinely retrieved to allow for a smear, frozen, and standard permanent pathologic analysis. It is helpful to pay attention to the directionality of the biopsy window and initially take the 2 specimens from different orientations based on the imaging characteristics. Should bleeding occur, steady irrigation should be performed with cool saline until the bleeding clears. Specimens are picked up immediately by the neuropathologist and reviewed with the operating neurosurgeon. Until a diagnostic result is obtained, the outer sheath of the needle should remain in place to facilitate additional biopsies if necessary.

Frameless Stereotactic Biopsy

Frameless neuronavigation techniques were introduced in the 1990s and have since evolved into a viable method of stereotactic biopsy in select circumstances.[13] The technology has been embraced by many neurosurgeons and is supplanting frame-based techniques in general neurosurgical practice. Briefly, a fine-cut MRI or CT scan is obtained and an intraoperative registration is achieved using either scalp fiducial markers or surface merging. These procedures are often performed under general anesthesia to eliminate any potential patient movement. The patients' head is fixed in a 3-point Mayfield clamp, and using a proprietary neuronavigation system, patients are registered, and the entry/target points are chosen in the same manner as previously described for frame-based procedures. Frameless neuronavigation technology is rapidly improving and advances, such as preregistered biopsy needles, navigation without rigid fixation, and novel systems with mechanical probe holders to maintain a fixed trajectory, are sure to improve the safety and efficacy of frameless stereotactic biopsies. However, because of the lengthy trajectories required for pineal region biopsies, the margin of error is generally greater for frameless compared with frame-based systems.

There are no studies that specifically examine the frameless stereotactic biopsy for pineal region lesions and, in fact, pineal region lesions are excluded from several series. Overall, the literature comparing frameless to frame-based biopsy would suggest that the safety and efficacy are comparable.[14–19] Smith and colleagues,[17] however, concluded that although equally efficacious, the frame-based approach required less anesthesia resources, less operating room time, and shorter hospital stays and should be considered the first-line approach for stereotactic brain biopsy. Lunsford and colleagues[20] report on their vast experience performing stereotactic biopsies and reaffirm the safety profile of frame-based biopsies and point out several significant advantages compared with frameless systems, including precise image integration, twist-drill access, preplotting of probe pathways, ability to use intravenous sedation without intubation, and a high degree of precision. They went on to compare their outcomes using frame-based biopsies with published outcomes using frameless approaches and demonstrated a 2.9% and 0.075% morbidity and mortality for frame-

based versus 8.6% and 1.5% for frameless systems. Thus, although frameless systems are available and have been gaining increased popularity, frame-based image-guided systems for pineal region biopsies are preferred because of their widespread availability, ease of use, and consistent accuracy.

Special Considerations in Children and Uncooperative Patients

Stereotactic procedures require specific modifications when performed in children. A primary limitation is the inability for most children to cooperate with the procedure. Many children are unable to tolerate application of the head frame. Thus, general anesthesia is typically required for children (and uncooperative or agitated adults) with intubation performed before the application of the CRW frame. The other consideration in children is the size and integrity of the skull. Infants often have incompletely ossified skulls, and dural or cortical penetration is a risk with overzealous pin tightening. Strict age or size cutoffs for use of the CRW system do not exist, but children with a head circumference of 25 cm or greater can be secured with pediatric pins and safely biopsied.[9]

Anesthetic Considerations

A successful pineal stereotactic biopsy depends on cooperation between surgeon, anesthesiologist, and patient. This relationship is facilitated by effective patient preparation regarding expectations and the nature of the procedure. These procedures are ideally performed with monitored anesthesia care using gentle amnestic sedation and generous local anesthesia, thus providing cooperative, comfortable, and safe patients. In the case of children or uncooperative patients, it may be necessary to use general anesthesia. This practice allows the use of muscle paralysis and absolutely still patients, thus, allowing safe passage of the biopsy needle. The use of general anesthesia, however, eliminates assessment of neurologic function and is associated with its own morbidity and mortality unrelated to the procedure. Critical attention to blood pressure management is also crucial to minimize the risks of hemorrhagic complications.[9]

Pathologic Considerations

Compared with open biopsy, image-guided stereotactic biopsy provides the advantage of obtaining tissue from a predetermined target within the lesion. The major disadvantage remains the small size of the biopsy cores, which may result in possible sampling error. This factor is especially true with pineal region lesions, which are often heterogeneous in nature. For instance, different degrees of malignancy may exist within regions of a pineal neoplasm resulting in an inaccurate diagnosis. Proper handling and interpretation of stereotactic biopsy specimens is crucial to deriving meaningful information and, thus, justifying the risks of the procedure.[10]

Biopsy specimens are placed in a petri dish with saline and are picked up immediately by the on-call neuropathologist.[9] The operating surgeon provides critical information concerning the clinical history, imaging characteristics, and consistency of the lesion. These factors must be taken into consideration to properly assess the cytologic features and correctly diagnose the lesion.[10] A smear is often prepared as the initial step in tissue processing. If a diagnosis can be rendered, the remainder of the tissue is fixed for permanent pathology.[9] If the smear is not diagnostic, a frozen section is typically performed. If a diagnosis still cannot be rendered, additional specimens may be requested. The decision to obtain additional specimens must take into account the reliability of the frozen specimen diagnosis, the risk of bleeding, and the likelihood of tumor heterogeneity.[8,10] A nondiagnostic specimen should prompt a reevaluation of the target and trajectory along with a reverification of the stereotactic coordinates. A firm lesion may be shifted by the end of the needle without actually penetrating the capsule and may require adjustment of the angle of trajectory or an increase in length. In some instances, the firmness of the tumor may not permit a specimen through the simple suction provided with a Nashold-type needle. A decision may be made to use a cup forceps or cutting biopsy needle to obtain the specimen. The surgeon must take into account the significantly increased risk of bleeding inherent in such a decision.

Perioperative Management

Standard neurosurgical care dictates the management of these patients, but a few critical points deserve mention. Within the first 24 hours postoperatively, patients are monitored in the neurologic intensive care unit and employ strict blood pressure control (systolic blood pressure less than 140 mmHg). Perioperative antibiotics are administered, but steroids or antiepileptics are not routinely used unless the clinical scenario dictates. Patients undergo immediate postoperative CT scans without contrast to rule out intracerebral hemorrhage and to establish a baseline should a neurologic deficit manifest itself. Patients are typically discharged in 24 to 48 hours postoperatively.[10]

LITERATURE REVIEW
Methods

An inclusive PubMed search performed for English-language articles published from 1990 to February 1, 2011, with the keywords pineal, tumor, region, biopsy, and stereotactic, returned 1001 articles. Of those, 60 articles were relevant to the biopsy of pineal tumors or the pineal region. Only those studies containing greater than 5 pineal region tumors represented in the article or in which pineal region tumors comprised greater than 10% of the patients/tumors in the study were included for analysis. Ultimately, 8 studies were analyzed and relevant data tallied into tabular format (**Table 1**). Mean percentage is provided when possible.

It is critical to keep in mind that reported series are based mostly on small numbers of patients, and, at best, retrospective data without adequate controls are available. Furthermore, the heterogeneity in technique, infrequent use of modern imaging modalities, and inconsistent reporting of complications make it difficult to draw any absolute conclusion regarding the safety/efficacy of stereotactic biopsy for pineal region tumors.

Diagnostic Accuracy

Determination of an accurate diagnosis is of paramount importance when performing a stereotactic biopsy. Because the procedure is not therapeutic, the goal should be reliable and reproducible tissue diagnosis; however, this is not always possible given the wide variety and inherent heterogeneity of these lesions. The mean diagnostic yield was 94.4% for stereotactic biopsy of the pineal region. This finding compares favorably when one looks at the stereotactic biopsies of other brain regions. Nevertheless, stereotactic biopsy provides minimal tissue sampling and can be prone to inaccuracies.[5,21] Only 1 study reliably looked at the diagnostic accuracy (ie, openly resected specimens confirming the stereotactic diagnosis). Konovalov and colleagues[22] demonstrated an 89% accuracy rate for the stereotactic biopsy of pineal region lesions. Given that this is a single study with significant bias (only 18 of the 61 biopsies were ever confirmed), it is difficult to provide a reliable estimate for the accuracy of stereotactic biopsy of the pineal region.

Morbidity and Mortality

The primary advantage of stereotactic biopsy is its minimally invasive nature, which is purported to provide a level of safety not afforded by open resection/biopsy. Certainly for individuals who could not withstand general anesthesia or a craniotomy,

Table 1
A summary of the eight studies which reviewed their experience with stereotactic pineal region biopsies since 1990. Diagnostic yield along with morbidity and mortality data are provided. Mean values are provided where appropriate

Authors	Year	Pineal/Total (%)	Frame Type	Needle	Trajectory	Diagnostic Yield (%)	Diagnostic Accuracy (%)	Mortality (%)	Major Morbidity (%)	Minor Morbidity (%)	Hemorrhage (%)
Popovic	1993	34/34 (100.0)	NR	NR	OA	33 (97.0)	NR	0	0	NR	NR
Dempsey	1992	15/15 (100.0)	NR	NR	OA, PL	13 (86.7)	NR	0	0	NR	1 (6.7)
Regis	1996	370/7885 (4.7)	T, L, O	S	OL, OA, PL	347 (93.8)	NR	5 (1.3)	3 (0.8)	27 (7.0)	16 (4.4)
Kreth	1996	106/106 (100.0)	R	F	OA, OL	103 (97.0)	NR	2 (1.9)	0 (0.0)	9 (8.5)	6 (5.7)
Sawin	1998	7/225 (3.1)	BRW, CRW	F, N	NR	NR	NR	0	0	1 (14.0)	1 (14.0)
Franzini	1997	20/20 (100.0)	L, CRW, O	NR	OA	20 (100.0)	NR	0 (0.0)	1 (5.0)	NR	NR
Field	2001	19/500 (3.8)	L	S, N	NR	NR	NR	0 (0.0)	0	0	4 (21.0)
Konovalov	2003	61/287 (21.3)	NR	NR	NR	56 (91.8)	16/18 (89.0)[a]	1 (1.6)	NR	NR	NR
Total		632/9072 (7.0)	—	—	—	572/606 (94.4)	—	8/632 (1.3)	4/571 (0.7)	37/502 (7.4)	28/552 (5.1)

Abbreviations: F, Forceps; L, Leksell; N, Nashold; NR, not reported; O, other; OA, oblique anterolateral; OL, orthogonal lateral; PL, posterolateral; R, Riechert; S, Sedan; T, Talairach.
[a] Only 18 patients underwent confirmatory open biopsy.

a stereotactic biopsy offers substantial advantages; however, there has been significant reluctance within the neurosurgical community to broadly use stereotactic biopsy in the pineal region given its proximity to critical vascular structures. The reviewed series demonstrate a low overall morbidity and mortality rate of 1%. The mortality rates ranged from 0.0% to 1.9% with a mean of 1.3%. Major morbidity was infrequent at 0.7% and minor morbidity occurred in 7.4% of patients.

Field and colleagues[23] concluded that stereotactic biopsy of the pineal region was associated with a nearly 5-fold increase in the risk of hemorrhage greater than 5 mm relative to all other locations. It is important to note, however, that none of the patients in this study experienced neurologic deficits secondary to these hemorrhages. Overall, the risk of hemorrhage associated with stereotactic biopsies of the pineal region is 5.1%, which is likely a more accurate estimate, and the clinical implication of small hemorrhage within this region remains to be defined.

When reviewing the diagnostic accuracy and associated morbidity of stereotactic biopsy in the pineal region, it is important to understand how these results compare with stereotactic biopsy elsewhere in the brain. The overall results of the pineal biopsies reviewed in this article are in line with larger series in the literature for stereotactic biopsies without consideration to location. In these series, the average morbidity and mortality rates were approximately 4% and the diagnostic yield was approximately 94%.[11,24]

All 5 cases of death in the study by Regis and colleagues[11] were performed via the orthogonal lateral trajectory, although statistical analysis in their study did not demonstrate a relationship between the choice of trajectory and the risk of morbidity. The risks of stereotactic biopsy must also be compared with those of open surgical biopsy or resection. Modern series of experienced surgeons indicate an approximately 4% mortality rate, with a morbidity rate between 3% and 12%.[3,8,25–27] Additionally, it is of interest to note the rare but possible risk of metastatic seeding along the biopsy tract with malignant tumors.[28]

SUMMARY

Modern neuroimaging techniques and advanced stereotactic guidance have helped make stereotactic biopsy a safe and efficacious means of obtaining a tissue diagnosis of pineal region tumors. Nevertheless, the heterogeneity of these lesions, perceived risk of stereotactic biopsy, and the potential benefit of surgical resection for benign lesions, and debulking before adjuvant therapy

continues to drive many surgeons toward open exploration. An unconditional policy of stereotactic biopsy as the initial management in all patients with pineal regions lesions is not reasonable, instead, the specifics of a clinical scenario should guide the diagnostic approach. Those patients with known primary systemic tumors, multiple lesions, invasive lesions where resection is not feasible, or with a medical condition that contraindicates an open procedure would be considered good candidates for a stereotactic biopsy.

REFERENCES

1. Araki C, Matsumoto S. Statistical reevaluation of pinealoma and related tumors in Japan. J Neurosurg 1969;30(2):146–9.
2. Poppen JL, Marino R Jr. Pinealomas and tumors of the posterior portion of the third ventricle. J Neurosurg 1968;28(4):357–64.
3. Bruce JN. Pineal tumors. In: Winn H, editor. Youman's neurological surgery. Philadelphia: WB Saunders Company; 2004. p. 1011–29.
4. Chapman PH, Linggood RM. The management of pineal area tumors: a recent reappraisal. Cancer 1980;46(5):1253–7.
5. Edwards MS, Hudgins RJ, Wilson CB, et al. Pineal region tumors in children. J Neurosurg 1988;68(5):689–97.
6. Jamieson KG. Excision of pineal tumors. J Neurosurg 1971;35(5):550–3.
7. Youssef AS, Keller JT, van Loveren HR. Novel application of computer-assisted cisternal endoscopy for the biopsy of pineal region tumors: cadaveric study. Acta Neurochir (Wien) 2007;149(4):399–406.
8. Bruce JN, Ogden AT. Surgical strategies for treating patients with pineal region tumors. J Neurooncol 2004;69(1–3):221–36.
9. Chen T, Lavine S, Amar A, et al. Stereotactic applications in third ventricular lesions. In: Apuzzo ML, editor. Surgery of the third ventricle. 2nd edition. Baltimore: Williams and Wilkins; 1998. p. 847–83.
10. Maciunas R. Stereotactic biopsy of pineal region lesions. In: Kaye A, Black P, editors. Operative neurosurgery. London: Churchill Livingstone; 2000. p. 841–5.
11. Regis J, Bouillot P, Rouby-Volot F, et al. Pineal region tumors and the role of stereotactic biopsy: review of the mortality, morbidity, and diagnostic rates in 370 cases. Neurosurgery 1996;39(5):907–12 [discussion: 912–4].
12. Dempsey PK, Kondziolka D, Lunsford LD. Stereotactic diagnosis and treatment of pineal region tumours and vascular malformations. Acta Neurochir (Wien) 1992;116(1):14–22.
13. Owen CM, Linskey ME. Frame-based stereotaxy in a frameless era: current capabilities, relative role,

and the positive- and negative predictive values of blood through the needle. J Neurooncol 2009;93(1): 139–49.

14. Dammers R, Haitsma IK, Schouten JW, et al. Safety and efficacy of frameless and frame-based intracranial biopsy techniques. Acta Neurochir (Wien) 2008; 150(1):23–9.

15. Dorward NL, Paleologos TS, Alberti O, et al. The advantages of frameless stereotactic biopsy over frame-based biopsy. Br J Neurosurg 2002;16(2):110–8.

16. Paleologos TS, Dorward NL, Wadley JP, et al. Clinical validation of true frameless stereotactic biopsy: analysis of the first 125 consecutive cases. Neurosurgery 2001;49(4):830–5 [discussion: 835–7].

17. Smith JS, Quinones-Hinojosa A, Barbaro NM, et al. Frame-based stereotactic biopsy remains an important diagnostic tool with distinct advantages over frameless stereotactic biopsy. J Neurooncol 2005; 73(2):173–9.

18. Woodworth G, McGirt MJ, Samdani A, et al. Accuracy of frameless and frame-based image-guided stereotactic brain biopsy in the diagnosis of glioma: comparison of biopsy and open resection specimen. Neurol Res 2005;27(4):358–62.

19. Woodworth GF, McGirt MJ, Samdani A, et al. Frameless image-guided stereotactic brain biopsy procedure: diagnostic yield, surgical morbidity, and comparison with the frame-based technique. J Neurosurg 2006; 104(2):233–7.

20. Lunsford LD, Niranjan A, Khan AA, et al. Establishing a benchmark for complications using frame-based stereotactic surgery. Stereotact Funct Neurosurg 2008;86(5):278–87.

21. Kraichoke S, Cosgrove M, Chandrasoma PT. Granulomatous inflammation in pineal germinoma. A cause of diagnostic failure at stereotaxic brain biopsy. Am J Surg Pathol 1988;12(9):655–60.

22. Konovalov AN, Pitskhelauri DI. Principles of treatment of the pineal region tumors. Surg Neurol 2003;59(4):250–68.

23. Field M, Witham TF, Flickinger JC, et al. Comprehensive assessment of hemorrhage risks and outcomes after stereotactic brain biopsy. J Neurosurg 2001; 94(4):545–51.

24. Ostertag CB, Mennel HD, Kiessling M. Stereotactic biopsy of brain tumors. Surg Neurol 1980;14(4): 275–83.

25. Bruce JN, Stein BM. Surgical management of pineal region tumors. Acta Neurochir (Wien) 1995;134(3–4): 130–5.

26. Jooma R, Kendall BE. Diagnosis and management of pineal tumors. J Neurosurg 1983;58(5):654–65.

27. Kreth FW, Schatz CR, Pagenstecher A, et al. Stereotactic management of lesions of the pineal region. Neurosurgery 1996;39(2):280–9 [discussion: 289–91].

28. Rosenfeld JV, Murphy MA, Chow CW. Implantation metastasis of pineoblastoma after stereotactic biopsy. Case report. J Neurosurg 1990;73(2):287–90.

Surgical Approaches to the Pineal Region

Benjamin C. Kennedy, MD[a],*, Jeffrey N. Bruce, MD[b]

KEYWORDS

• Pineal region • Pineal tumors • Resection • Surgery

Surgical strategy for pineal region tumors is affected not only by anatomic considerations but by pathologic features as well. The varied pathologies that occur in this region can dictate a range of surgical strategies from gross total resection or debulking to biopsy or medical management.

HISTORY OF PINEAL REGION SURGERY

Since its birth in the early twentieth century, surgery of the pineal region has matured, reflecting an understanding of the region's varied pathologies as well as evolution of surgical technologies and techniques, creating a modern, nuanced, multidisciplinary approach to these tumors.

Among the earliest descriptions of operative approaches to pineal tumors, published in 1913, were interhemispheric transcallosal, an approach modified by Dandy in the 1920s.[1,2] Pineal tumor surgery in the 1910s through the early 1930s was dangerous for a multitude of reasons beyond the anatomic challenges, including the lack of experience, operative microscope, and adequate lighting.[3,4] In 1931, Van Wagenen[5] introduced a transcortical transventricular approach through the right parietal lobe and right lateral ventricle. Horrax[6] reported a variation on Dandy's approach involving resection of the occipital lobe to afford better exposure of large tumors. Through the 1940s and 1950s, use of these and Dandy's original approach did little to improve outcomes for these patients, with perioperative mortality of 20% to 70%.

In the 1960s, Poppen first described the occipital transtentorial approach, though during this same period radiotherapy became the first-line treatment, as these patients fared better than surgery patients in the aggregate. However, as only half of pineal tumors are radiosensitive,[7] at least half of all pineal tumor patients received unnecessary whole brain radiation, particularly those with benign or low-grade lesions, who should have the best prognosis. The need for tissue diagnosis thus became clear, and a modern pathology-driven management strategy was born. Stein's infratentorial supracerebellar approach adapted from Krause[8] and Jamieson's experience with Poppen's approach,[9] both published in 1971 and using the operative microscope, ushered in the modern era of safer radical pineal surgery, and allowed the effective treatment of all types of pineal pathology.

The 1970s also saw reports of stereotactic biopsy,[10] stereotactic radiosurgery,[11] and endoscopic biopsy of pineal tumors, a practice that became commonplace by the 1990s, often coupled with endoscopic third ventriculostomy for treatment of hydrocephalus.

INDICATIONS FOR SURGERY

The pineal region produces an unrivaled variety of neoplastic and nonneoplastic masses, half of which are radiosensitive.[7] Therefore, indication for surgical management of pineal tumors depends on tumor markers, pathologic findings on biopsy, and the degree and chronicity of associated hydrocephalus. Contrast magnetic resonance imaging (MRI) is indicated prior to any nonurgent management, but does not reliably differentiate among histologic subtypes; its utility is thus to plan the operative approach, identify the relationships between the tumor and other anatomic structures, and determine whether total resection can be attempted safely.

[a] Department of Neurological Surgery, Columbia University, 710 West 168th Street, New York, NY 10032, USA
[b] Department of Neurological Surgery, Columbia University College of Physicians and Surgeons, Room 434, Neurological Institute, Columbia University Medical Center, 710 West 168th Street, New York, NY 10032, USA
* Corresponding author.
E-mail address: benjamin.c.kennedy@gmail.com

Neurosurg Clin N Am 22 (2011) 367–380
doi:10.1016/j.nec.2011.05.007
1042-3680/11/$ – see front matter © 2011 Elsevier Inc. All rights reserved.

Tumor Markers

Considering the attendant morbidity of pineal region surgery or even biopsy, noninvasive means of obtaining an accurate diagnosis of a radiosensitive tumor should always be attempted. Detection of β-human chorionic gonadotropin (β-HCG) or α-fetoprotein, or both, in the serum or cerebrospinal fluid (CSF) suggests a malignant germ cell tumor and is an indication for radiotherapy and chemotherapy without resection or biopsy, though management of hydrocephalus is still usually warranted.[12] CSF can be obtained during external ventricular drain placement, endoscopic third ventriculostomy, shunting, or via low-volume lumbar puncture. It must be noted that pineal masses cause obstructive hydrocephalus, and lumbar puncture in this setting could precipitate herniation.

Hydrocephalus Management

Most patients with pineal region tumors present with hydrocephalus, and in their preoperative evaluation, the acuity of the situation is primarily dictated by the degree of hydrocephalus and clinical presentation. If urgent, bedside placement of a temporizing external ventricular drain can be performed until definitive treatment strategy is determined. In the event of subsequent resection, some patients may not require continued CSF diversion. This strategy can be employed in nonurgent cases as well, particularly in the setting of mild hydrocephalus with a simple cyst or well-encapsulated tumor.

Optimal surgical strategy usually involves endoscopic third ventriculostomy, as these tumors create an obstructive hydrocephalus, and some can be biopsied through the posterior third ventricle during the same procedure, if indicated.[13,14] The procedure is safe and effective, and is preferred over ventriculoperitoneal shunting unless tumor occupies the floor of the third ventricle, or mass effect distorts anatomy thus making the relationship of the basilar artery with the floor of the third ventricle unfavorable. Ventriculoperitoneal shunting is also an acceptable means of CSF diversion, though it is associated with higher rates of infection, malfunction, overshunting, subdural hematoma, and peritoneal metastasis.

Biopsy Versus Resection

The decision between biopsy alone or resection should take into account the treatment objectives as well as the risks of each of the possible procedures. The primary objective in the surgical management of pineal region tumors is to establish accurate pathologic diagnosis, which dictates further surgical strategy, adjuvant therapy, metastatic workup, prognosis, and follow-up plans.[13,15–24] The secondary objective is resection, whether partial or complete.

Considering the diversity of histologic findings in pineal masses, in the absence of positive tumor markers accurate tissue diagnosis is essential. The most reliable strategy for accurate diagnosis is adequate tissue sampling, which is limited in stereotactic and endoscopic biopsy, and much more feasible in open procedures.[17,25]

A major advantage of open microsurgical techniques is resection. Approximately one-third of pineal tumors are benign, and resection affords the best opportunity for long-term recurrence-free survival.[15,20,24,26–28] For malignant tumors, the clinical impact of maximal tumor resection is less well documented, though several reports have correlated extent of tumor resection with improved response to adjuvant therapy and increased survival.[28–35] Other advantages of more aggressive resection include the potential to control hydrocephalus without a second procedure and reduced risk of postoperative hemorrhage into residual tumor bed.

These advantages of open surgery are contingent on avoidance of complications. Favorable results are achievable, but are considerably dependent on the experience and judgment of the surgeon, beyond what is typically necessary for an intracranial tumor operation.[13] Indeed, the risk-benefit balance may shift depending on the surgeon as much as the anatomy.[15]

The primary advantage of stereotactic biopsy over open microsurgical tissue sampling is that the stereotactic procedure carries a lower morbidity through limited invasiveness and ability to avoid general anesthesia. However, the deep venous system, choroidal arteries, and multiple pial surfaces to be traversed during the procedure, as well as limited ability of nearby brain to tamponade even minor bleeding, makes this area among the most hazardous in the brain for stereotactic biopsy.

Endoscopic biopsy of pineal tumors through the ventricles has been reported as an alternative method for securing a tissue diagnosis.[36–42] In addition to sampling error, a major drawback of this procedure is that the tumor is biopsied along its ventricular surface, where there is no tissue turgor to tamponade the bleeding. Even minor bleeding within the CSF space can be difficult to manage, a problem that is compounded by the highly vascular properties of many pineal tumors. This procedure typically is combined with a ventriculostomy. However, even with flexible endoscopes it is difficult to perform a biopsy simultaneously with a ventriculostomy because the trajectory required is different for each procedure. The rigid endoscope is not easily maneuverable without risk of damage to the fornix and the septal and thalamostriate veins at the foramen of Monro. A suitable entry point through the forehead might allow the use of a rigid scope, but this offers no advantage over a simple stereotactic biopsy. More typically, endoscopes have been used to aspirate pineal cysts; however, the benefits of this approach are equivocal.

SURGICAL APPROACHES
Operative Procedures

Several variations on approaches to the pineal region exist, but essentially they are categorized as supratentorial or infratentorial.[13,24,43,44] Supratentorial approaches include transcallosal interhemispheric, occipital transtentorial, and the rarely used transcortical transventricular.[5,20,43,45] The infratentorial approach is through a natural corridor created between the tentorium and the cerebellum (**Fig. 1**).[8,46] Many of these approaches are interchangeable, although the surgeon's experience and several anatomic caveats play a role in the choice of approach. Supratentorial approaches afford greater exposure than do infratentorial approaches, allowing access to large tumors that extend supratentorially or laterally to the trigone, but they have the disadvantage of forcing the surgeon to work around the convergence of the vein of Galen and internal cerebral veins. The midline infratentorial location of most pineal tumors gives the infratentorial supracerebellar approach several natural advantages.[43,47] It is performed with the patient in the sitting position, whereby gravity allows the cerebellum and the tumor to drop downward. As the deep venous system is dorsal to pineal tumors, it and the velum interpositum can easily be dissected off the tumor by this approach. With appropriate extra-long instruments, even tumors extending anteriorly into the third ventricle can be removed.

Patient Positioning

Numerous patient positions have been described for these approaches, each having advantages and disadvantages.

Sitting position
The sitting position is usually preferred for the infratentorial supracerebellar approach.[43,47] Gravity works in the surgeon's favor by reducing pooling of blood in the operative field and by facilitating dissection of the tumor from the deep venous system. The risks for air embolism, pneumocephalus, or subdural hematoma associated with cortical collapse can be anticipated and managed with proper precautions.[43,48] Precordial Doppler monitoring or a drop in end-tidal CO_2 can detect air emboli, and a central venous catheter can be used to remove entrapped air if necessary. Optimization of the sitting position involves lowering the table to the floor and bringing the patient to position by manipulating the table. The head is flexed

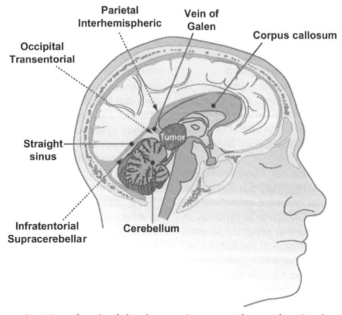

Fig. 1. The approximate direction of each of the three major approaches to the pineal region.

so that the tentorium is approximately parallel to the floor. At least 2 fingerbreadths of space are needed between the patient's chin and sternum to avoid compromising the airway and venous return. The patient's legs should be elevated to assist venous return. A 3-point vise type of head holder keeps the head immobile.

Lateral position

The lateral decubitus position with the dependent, nondominant right hemisphere down is another useful approach.[49] The head is raised approximately 30° above the horizontal in the midsagittal plane, especially for the transcallosal approach. For the occipital transtentorial approach, the head should be positioned with the patient's nose rotated 30° toward the floor, or the three-quarter prone position can be used, which is essentially an extension of the lateral position except that the head is at an oblique 45° angle with the nondominant hemisphere dependent.[50] The nondominant hemisphere is easily retracted with the help of gravity. Surgeon fatigue is reduced because the surgeon's hands are not extended to the degree they are with patients in the sitting position.

Prone position

The prone position is simple and safe for supratentorial approaches, and is generally comfortable for the surgeon[43,45] but can be cumbersome for the infratentorial approach. This position is useful when two surgeons work together through an operative microscope and is often useful in the pediatric population. When desired for infratentorial approaches in infants, the position of the head can be rotated 15° away from the craniotomy side in a variation known as the Concorde position.

Operative Approaches

Infratentorial supracerebellar approach

The infratentorial supracerebellar approach is usually performed with the patient in the sitting position.[24,43,47] If necessary, a ventricular drain can be placed in the trigone of the lateral ventricle through a burr hole in the midpupillary line at the lambdoid suture.

A suboccipital exposure is begun through a linear midline incision extending from just above the torcular and external occipital protuberance down to the level of the C4 spinous process. A single low-profile, self-retaining retractor is used to retract the muscles and fascia of the suboccipital region for exposure of the suboccipital bone. The craniotomy is centered just below the torcular. The bony opening must be sufficient to provide access for the surgical instruments and adequate light from the operating microscope.

A craniotomy is preferred over a craniectomy because it reduces the incidence of postoperative aseptic meningitis, fluid collections, and discomfort. Slots are drilled over the sagittal sinus, above the torcular, over both transverse sinuses, and approximately 1 or 2 cm above the foramen magnum in the midline. A craniotome is used to connect the slots. Sufficient bone should be removed above the transverse sinus to ensure that the view along the tentorium is not obscured. Any bone edges should be carefully waxed, and all venous bleeding should be controlled to avoid air emboli.

The dura is opened in a semilunar curve extending from the lateral aspects of the exposure and reflected upward on slight tension. If the posterior fossa is tight, fluid can be removed from a ventricular drain or by opening the cisterna magna.

To open the infratentorial corridor, the arachnoid adhesions and midline bridging veins between the dorsal surface of the cerebellum and the tentorium are cauterized and carefully divided, preserving any veins found laterally.[51] Cauterizing the bridging veins and dividing them midway can minimize the nuisance of bleeding from the sinus. The cerebellum then drops away from the tentorium to provide an excellent corridor with minimal brain retraction. Additional adhesions and bridging veins can be divided when they become visible near the anterior vermis as the cerebellum is retracted. With the retractor in place, the opalescent arachnoid covering the pineal region can be seen. The operating microscope is brought in at this time.

Under the microscope, the arachnoid overlying the quadrigeminal plate is sharply opened; this is generally an avascular plane, and minimal cautery is necessary. The precentral cerebellar vein is identified as it courses from the anterior vermis to the vein of Galen and should be carefully dissected, cauterized, and divided (**Fig. 2**). Although this vein can be taken without difficulty, it is not advisable to cauterize any other veins of the deep venous system. With the posterior surface of the tumor exposed, the central portion is cauterized and opened with a long-handled knife or bayonet scissors. Specimens can be taken from within the capsule and sent for frozen diagnosis.

The tumor is then internally debulked with a variety of instruments such as suction, cautery, tumor forceps, and a Cavitron ultrasonic aspirator if necessary. Most tumors are soft and can generally be suctioned with a large-bore Japanese-style suction device with variable control. As the tumor is decompressed, the capsule can be separated from the surrounding thalamus. Most of the vessels along the wall of the capsule are choroidal

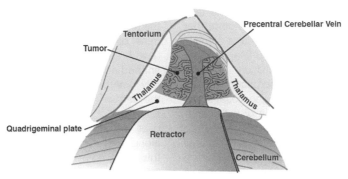

Fig. 2. Microscopic view during an infratentorial supracerebellar approach. The patient is in the sitting position, the cerebellum is retracted inferiorly, and the precentral cerebellar vein runs between the surgeon and the tumor.

vessels and need not be preserved. The dissection continues until the third ventricle is encountered. The tumor is then carefully dissected inferiorly off the brainstem. This stage is often the most difficult of the tumor dissection, and can be facilitated by retracting the tumor superiorly and dissecting it bluntly off the brainstem under direct vision. Finally, the tumor is removed superiorly after separating the attachments along the velum interpositum and the deep venous system. Flexible mirrors can be useful for examining the inferior portion of the tumor bed to verify the extent of resection and to avoid leaving any blood clots. **Fig. 3** depicts preoperative and postoperative MRI scans from a patient with a tumor suited for this approach.

Transcallosal interhemispheric approach

This approach between the falx and hemisphere of the brain involves a corridor along the parieto-occipital junction. Any of the previously described patient positions can be used for this approach, although the prone or sitting position is generally preferred. Positioning of the bone flap depends on where the tumor is centered in the third ventricle.[45,52,53] A U-shaped scalp flap extending across the midline and reflected laterally followed by a wide craniotomy roughly 8 cm in length generally over the vertex provides flexibility in determining the corridor and avoiding bridging veins whenever possible. The craniotomy should extend 1 to 2 cm to the left of the sagittal sinus.

The dura is opened in U-shaped fashion and reflected medially toward the sagittal sinus. The bridging veins are inspected, and an approach is chosen that will minimize the number of veins sacrificed. It is unlikely that sufficient exposure can be achieved without sacrificing at least one bridging vein, although sacrifice of more than one should be avoided if possible. Because these tumors are deeply seated, even a small opening provides a wide angle of deep exposure. The

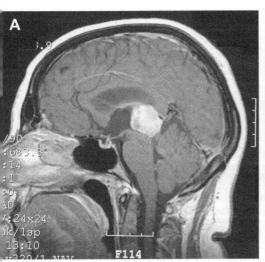
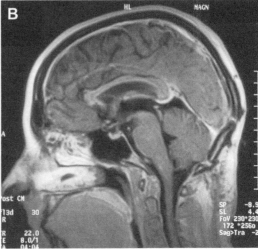

Fig. 3. (*A*) Preoperative magnetic resonance image (MRI) from a patient with a pineal tumor amenable to resection via the supracerebellar-infratentorial approach. (*B*) Postoperative MRI demonstrating gross total resection.

parietal lobe is gently retracted, as is the falx, which may be divided inferiorly to provide further retraction; this is generally a nonvascular corridor with few adhesions between the falx and the cingulate gyrus. The corpus callosum is easily identified with the operating microscope by its striking white appearance. The pericallosal arteries are retracted either to one side or with separate retractors to each side. The opening into the corpus callosum, centered over the maximal bulge of the tumor, is generally about 2 cm, which is not likely to lead to disconnection syndrome or cognitive impairment. Even more posterior openings in the splenium have been performed routinely without deficits. The corpus callosum is generally thin and can be opened with gentle suction and cautery. The lateral extent of the opening is determined by the amount that is sufficient to expose the tumor and avoid damage to the pericallosal arteries. If necessary, the tentorium and falx can be divided to provide additional exposure.

Once through the corpus callosum, the dorsal surface of the tumor can be seen, and the veins of the deep venous system must be identified. Whether one vein can be sacrificed safely is questionable, but certainly interruption of two would have a devastating result. Once the tumor is exposed, it is debulked and then dissected as described previously. Leaving a ventricular drain in place for 1 or 2 days is optional.

Occipital transtentorial approach

A three-quarter prone position is generally preferred for the occipital transtentorial approach. Although some find orientation difficult intraoperatively, stereotactic guidance can be helpful. By dividing the tentorium, excellent exposure of the quadrigeminal plate is achieved, thus making it particularly useful for tumors that extend inferiorly. A U-shaped right occipital scalp flap is reflected inferiorly, with the medial vertical limb beginning just to the left of midline at about the level of the torcular.[20,46,53] A burr hole is placed in the midline over the sagittal sinus just above the torcular, along with another burr hole 6 to 10 cm above this, followed by a generous craniotomy extending 1 to 2 cm left of midline. Gravity helps with retraction of the nondominant occipital lobe, which is also facilitated by the lack of bridging veins near the occipital pole. Mannitol and ventricular drainage are useful for relaxing the brain and minimizing the risk for hemianopsia from excessive occipital lobe retraction.

Under the operating microscope, the straight sinus is identified so that the tentorium can be divided adjacent to it. A retractor can be placed over the falx for exposure. The inferior sagittal sinus and falx can be divided to facilitate further falcine retraction (**Fig. 4**). At this point, the arachnoid overlying the tumor and the quadrigeminal cisterns can be seen. Tumor removal proceeds as described earlier while taking care to avoid injury to the deep venous system. **Fig. 5** depicts preoperative and postoperative MRI scans from a patient with a tumor suited for this approach.

Transcortical transventricular approach

This approach is rarely used because the exposure is limited and the need for a cortical incision is undesirable. Of course, an entry point should be chosen in noneloquent cortex. Stereotactic

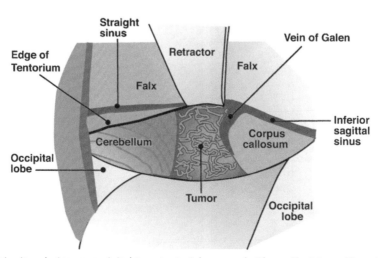

Fig. 4. Microscopic view during an occipital transtentorial approach. The patient is positioned right ear down, with gravity assisting the retraction of the right occipital lobe downward. The free edge of the tentorium has been cut to the right of the straight sinus, exposing the tumor and cerebellum.

A

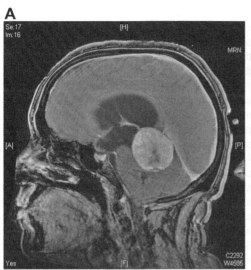

B

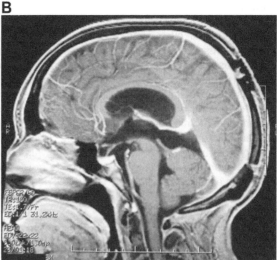

Fig. 5. (*A*) Preoperative MRI from a patient with a large pineal region tumor with significant caudal extension. Such tumors are best removed through an occipital transtentorial approach. (*B*) Postoperative MRI following removal via the occipital transtentorial approach.

guidance is often useful with this approach and may be desirable for a tumor that extends into the lateral ventricle.

Postoperative Care

High-dose steroids should be maintained for the first few days and then tapered as the patient's condition improves.[46,53] Lethargy and mild cognitive impairment are common and make it difficult to evaluate neurologic status in the immediate postoperative period, particularly in patients with extensive subdural air as a result of the sitting position. Careful and frequent neurologic examinations are necessary, and any changes should be investigated by computed tomography to rule out the possibility of hydrocephalus, hemorrhage, or residual air. Shunt malfunction is a frequent immediate problem caused by air, blood, or operative debris; it is particularly worrisome because deterioration and major morbidity can occur rapidly.

Patients should be encouraged to mobilize and ambulate as early as possible in the postoperative period. With ataxic patients, physical therapy and rehabilitation consultation are important to support rapid mobilization.

If a drain was placed at the time of surgery, it should be removed or converted to a shunt within the first 72 hours to minimize the risk for infection. Postoperative MRI with gadolinium enhancement should be performed within 72 hours to determine the extent of resection and to guide future management decisions.

ROLE OF SURGICAL RESECTION BY HISTOLOGY

The effectiveness of debulking of pineal tumors is pathology dependent. The greatest benefit occurs in the context of benign or low-grade tumors, whereas the effect of debulking of higher grade is more dependent on the effectiveness of adjuvant therapies. The analysis of the impact of surgery on outcome for these tumors is further complicated by the continuing development of improved therapies and treatment strategies, long-term survival with inadequate follow-up, inadequate assessment of degree of resection, small numbers of cases of each specific pathology, historical inaccuracies in establishing definitive diagnoses, and retrospective design of most studies.

Despite these issues, there are clear and consistent trends that demonstrate the benefits of aggressive surgery. To extrapolate these findings into a definitive mandate for open surgery for all patients would be premature, as none of the studies provide a suitable direct comparison with radiosurgery. It is possible that favorable outcomes correlate most strongly with tumor histology and still undefined biologic characteristics rather than with specific treatment modalities. At present, series describing surgical resection have the benefit of larger numbers of patients and longer follow-up than studies involving radiosurgery.

Benign Pineal Region Tumors

Benign pathology accounts for approximately one-third of pineal region lesions and is clearly associated with excellent prognosis.[15,43,54,55] These lesions include meningiomas, epidermoids, teratomas, pineal cysts, and pilocytic astrocytomas. Aggressive surgical treatment with the goal of gross total resection invariably results in long-term remission and potential cure. In addition, this group of patients has the lowest incidence of operative complications. Pineal cysts are normal anatomic variants of the pineal gland and generally do not warrant intervention. When causing obstructive hydrocephalus or showing evidence of progression, surgical resection is indicated, with excellent results.[56]

Germinomas

Germinomas, the most common tumor in this region, are highly radiosensitive with expectations of 80% to 90% long-term survival when adequate (>5500 cGy) radiation doses are given to the tumor and surrounding ventricles.[30,57] This success can be misleading, as up to 20% of germinomas produce fatal metastases, many despite radiographic cures.[58–61] A small percentage of pure germinomas are associated with slightly elevated β-HCG levels, a finding correlating with a less favorable prognosis. To reduce serious cognitive and endocrinological morbidity from whole brain radiation, especially in the pediatric population, investigators have sought other therapeutic options including chemotherapy and stereotactic radiosurgery. Other trials currently employ stereotactic radiosurgery and chemotherapy as a first-line therapy, reserving whole brain radiation for nonresponders.

The proven success of adjuvant therapy for germinomas has decreased the emphasis on debulking. Some investigators support limited resection, based primarily on a series of 29 patients with intracranial germinomas achieving a 100% survival rate with adjuvant therapy at a median follow-up of 42 months regardless of degree of resection.[59] However, this series is not straightforward because only 10 patients had solitary pineal tumors (8 with gross total resection), and it is possible that longer follow-up periods would have demonstrated survival differences.

Contrary evidence is provided by an analysis of the International CNS Germ Cell Tumor Study, which observed a trend toward improved survival with radical resection in 8 patients who underwent chemotherapy alone.[35] Alternative explanations may involve survival bias within the radical resection group, due to favorable biological tumor characteristics associated with resectability or the reduced sampling error in the radical resection group minimizing the possibility of undetected

teratoma or nongerminomatous malignant germ cell tumors. Although the benefits of resection are debatable with germinomas, few would question the wisdom of securing a biopsy-proved diagnosis.

The exquisite radiosensitivity of germinomas was responsible for the now obsolete strategy of empiric radiation therapy without biopsy, which prevailed in the pre-microsurgery era. This strategy is still followed in certain areas of East Asia where germinomas account for up to 50% of all pineal tumors and up to 85% of pineal masses in male patients between the ages of 15 and 35 years.[62,63] However, given the proven safety of both biopsy and open surgery, treatment without tissue diagnosis is difficult to justify. Studies have demonstrated up to a 26% increase in 5-year postradiation survival among histologically confirmed germinomas compared with unbiopsied tumors assumed to be germinomas.[64] Many of such so-called germinomas are in fact teratomas, which are radioresistant, whereas others consist of mixed tumors with nongerminomatous elements that might respond to radiation but still require adjuvant chemotherapy for optimal long-term survival.

Nongerminomatous Germ Cell Tumors

The nongerminomatous malignant germ cell tumors, including endodermal sinus tumors, choriocarcinomas, and embryonal carcinomas, carry a poor prognosis. Most are diagnosed on the basis of elevated β-HCG or α-fetoprotein levels, which make biopsy unnecessary, although these tumors can occur without elevated markers.

Nongerminomatous malignant germ cell tumors are radiosensitive, with optimal outcomes occurring when radiation is combined with chemotherapy. Their rarity and propensity toward mixed pathology have made their management and accurate assessment of their natural history difficult to evaluate. Clinical trials have used radical surgery alternatively as a primary intervention followed by adjuvant chemotherapy and radiation,[65–67] or in a "second-look" capacity for persistent lesions on MRI following adjuvant therapy and the normalization of CSF markers.[68–70] Studies have indicated the beneficial effects of radical resection including at least one report with statistical significance,[33] but in most analyses benefits from radical surgery have been either anecdotal or not statistically significant.[30,35]

Nevertheless, the best outcomes appear to have come from the second-look trials, and excellent analyses of the surgical arms of these trials are instructive.[71,72] Open surgery has a role in second-look surgery, which is performed when a residual mass is present following radiation and chemotherapy. Using this strategy, 5-year survival rates of 90% have been achieved, a remarkable improvement from the less than 2-year median survival reported in the early 1990s.[24,70] If present, residual tumor invariably represents benign germ cell elements that are not sensitive to these treatments and therefore surgery provides the optimal treatment. The second look is also helpful diagnostically, as malignant elements in residual tumors indicate the need for further chemotherapy.

Pineal Parenchymal Tumors

Pineal parenchymal tumors exist along a continuum from the essentially benign pineocytoma to the aggressively malignant pineoblastoma. Intermediate-grade pineal parenchymal tumors have been termed pineal parenchymal tumors of intermediate differentiation, mixed pineocytoma/pineoblastoma, or pineocytoma with anaplasia,[29] and a grading system that predicts prognosis continues to evolve.[73] Pineal parenchymal tumors are rare, and treatment varies dramatically according to pathology. As with other pineal region tumors, accurate tissue diagnosis is essential before initiating therapy. Although "clinicopathologic" studies have analyzed clinical courses of pineal parenchymal tumors in aggregate,[18,31] assessing the role of surgery for these lesions requires establishing categories based on pathology and patient age. Not only do these tumors behave differently based on pathology, but tumors of similar pathology behave differently according to patient age.

Pineocytomas are indolent tumors, optimally treated by radical surgery alone, and their prognosis and management parallels those of benign pineal region tumors. Exceptions to this rule may be pediatric cases of pineocytoma, which may behave more aggressively. In adults, surgical resection with or without radiation therapy is associated with complete long-term remission.[28,34]

Aggressive and prone to metastasis, pineoblastomas are histologically identical to primitive neuroectodermal tumors (PNET), and have historically been treated with radical surgery as well as adjuvant radiation and/or chemotherapy.[74] Like other PNETs, pineoblastomas carry a much worse prognosis in the pediatric population than in adults. Pineocytomas and intermediate-grade/mixed lesions are rare in children, whereas pineocytomas are the most common pineal parenchymal tumor in adults. Given the difference in behavior and distribution between pediatric and adult pineal parenchymal tumors, most investigators attempt to treat and analyze these two groups separately.

Although some investigators have advocated treatment of pediatric pineoblastoma with radiation alone, others have followed the lessons from treatment of the more common posterior fossa PNETs whose prognosis is intimately tied to the extent of surgical resection.[75] Clinical trials of PNETs (both pineal and nonpineal) have universally advocated gross total resection and have focused on developing chemotherapy regimens to reduce effective doses of radiation in children older than 4 years,[32,76–78] as well as to bridge the gap between diagnosis and reach a radiation-tolerant age in younger patients.[77,79] Objective assessments of the effect of extent of resection have shown trends toward better outcomes with radical surgery, but fall short of significance because of small cohort sizes.[31,32]

In adults with malignant pineal parenchymal tumors, long-term remission is not unusual and aggressive surgical resection seems beneficial. In a multicenter, retrospective review of 101 cases, 56 patients received surgery followed by radiation and/or chemotherapy and 44 were treated primarily with radiotherapy after diagnostic biopsy.[29] Numerous cases of tumor control were achieved by both general strategies, although patients undergoing surgery were twice as likely to be tumor-free as patients who received radiation alone. The study was unable to analyze the degree of surgical resection; however, the absence of residual tumor following treatment resulted in 100% 10-year survival, a finding that indirectly supports radical surgical resection. This study also demonstrates the prognostic importance of accurate tissue sampling through open surgery, as median survival for pineoblastoma patients was 77 months compared with 165 months for patients with tumors of intermediate differentiation.

Pineal Region Astrocytomas

Few reports specifically discuss pineal region astrocytomas, which include tumors arising from astrocytes within the pineal gland, brainstem, or thalamus. Astrocytomas arising in the pineal gland are often cystic, and complete surgical resection is achievable, resulting in probable cure.[24,26] Among astrocytomas of the quadrigeminal plate, the role of surgery is not clearly defined, and there is evidence that these tumors frequently follow an indolent natural history.[80]

OUTCOME

Due to the operating microscope, as well as advancements in surgical technique, neuroanesthesia, and postoperative care, the modern era has seen outcomes from radical surgery improve

Table 1
Outcomes of surgical resection in the modern era

Study	Year	No. of Cases	Approach	Patient Population	Pathology	GTR (%)	Mortality (%)	Major Morbidity (%)	Permanent Minor Morbidity (%)
Hoffman et al[81]	1983	61	TC/SCIT	Peds	All	NA	20[a]	NA	NA
Neuwelt[21]	1985	13	OTT	Adult/Peds	All	60	0	0	20
Lapras et al[20]	1987	86	TC/OTT	Adult/Peds	All	65	5.8[b]	5.8	28
Edwards et al[17]	1988	36	TT/OTT/SCIT	Peds	All	NA	0	3.3	3.3
Pluchino et al[22]	1989	40	SCIT	Adult/Peds	All	25	5	NA	NA
Luo et al[82]	1989	64	OTT	Adult/Peds	All	21	10	NA	NA
Vaquero et al[28]	1992	29	TC/SCIT/OTT	Adult/Peds	All	NA	11	NA	NA
Herrmann et al[83]	1992	49	IHTC/SCIT	Adult/Peds	All	NA	8	NA	NA
Bruce and Stein[15,46]	1995	160	SCIT/TC/OTT	Adult/Peds	All	45	4	3	19
Chandy and Damaraju[55]	1998	48	SCIT/OTT	Adult/Peds	"Benign lesions"	55	0	NA	NA
Kang et al[84]	1998	16	OTT/SCIT/TC	Adult/Peds	All	37.5	0	0	19
Shin et al[85]	1998	21	OTT	Adult/Peds	All	54.5	0	0	5
Konovalov and Pitskhelauvri[19]	2003	201	OTT (54%), SCIT (34%)	Adult/Peds	All	58	10[c]	NA	>20
Bruce[13]	2004	81	SCIT/TC/OTT	Adult/Peds	All	47	1	2	NA
Jia[86]	2011	150	TCIF	Peds	All	86	0	NA	NA

Abbreviations: GTR, patients with gross total resection; IHTC, interhemispheric transcallosal; NA, not available; OTT, occipital transtentorial; Peds, pediatric; SCIT, supracerebellar infratentorial; TC, transcallosal; TCIF, transcallosal interforniceal.

[a] All except one mortality prior to 1975.

[b] Combined major morbidity/mortality reduced to 2.8% in last 40 patients.

[c] Mortality rate of 1.8% in the 168 resections after 1990.

considerably. The results of modern series are listed in **Table 1**, and report perioperative mortality from radical resection of 0% to 11%, major morbidity of 3% to 6.8%, and permanent minor morbidity of 3% to 28%. Of note, the higher complication rates are from the older series, and recent operative mortality rates are 0% to 2%.

The most serious complications from pineal surgery involve postoperative hemorrhage, most commonly from malignant, vascular tumors that have been incompletely resected, sometimes after several days.[13,46] Extraocular movement dysfunction, papillary abnormalities, and ataxia are potential sequelae related to brainstem and cerebellar manipulation. These problems tend to be temporary and reversible over periods ranging from days to up to 1 year. Similarly, cognitive impairment is usually transient and is likely related to intracranial air or manipulation around the third ventricle. Increased severity and incidence of complications correlates with prior radiation, invasive/malignant tumors, and presence of preoperative symptoms.[13,24,46] Complications from hemispheric manipulation are unique to the supratentorial approaches.[24] Visual field disturbances, usually reversible, can occur with the occipital approach. Hemiparesis or sensory deficits may accompany the parietal interhemispheric approach, resulting from brain retraction or venous compromise from sacrifice of bridging veins. Of course, these risks must be weighed against the benefits of surgical resection, including (1) the potential for cure with benign or low-grade lesions, (2) increased efficacy of adjuvant therapies and improved survival with higher-grade lesions, (3) improvement of symptoms from mass effect, (4) the potential for avoidance of side effects of radiation or chemotherapy, and rarely, (5) the improvement or prevention of hydrocephalus and the risks associated with its management.

SUMMARY

The pineal region can harbor highly diverse histologic tumor subtypes. Because optimal therapeutic strategies vary with tumor type, an accurate diagnosis is the foundation of enlightened management decisions. Either stereotactic biopsy or open surgery is essential for securing tissue for pathologic examination. Biopsy has the advantage of ease and minimal invasiveness, but is associated with more sampling errors than open surgery. The emergence of endoscopic techniques and stereotactic radiosurgery provide complementary options to improve pineal tumor management

and will assume greater importance in the neurosurgeon's armamentarium.

Aggressive surgical resection has clearly improved the outcome for benign, low-grade, and even some malignant tumors. The benefits of resection for malignant germ cell tumors and some malignant pineal cell tumors are less clearly defined, but are likely beneficial if achieved without significant morbidity. Improvements in surgical techniques along with improved neuroanesthesia and postoperative care in the intensive care unit have combined to reduce surgical morbidity and justify increasingly aggressive approaches. These techniques are sophisticated, and require experience and sound judgment to achieve the maximal benefits. The evolution of newer techniques including endoscopy and stereotactic radiosurgery means that the future for patients with pineal tumors will be increasingly optimistic.

ACKNOWLEDGMENTS

We greatly appreciate Trine Giaever for her original illustrations.

REFERENCES

1. Oppenheim H, Krause F. [Operative Erfolge bei Geschwulsten der sehhugelund Vierbugelgegend]. Berl Klin Wochenschr 1913;50:2316 [in German].
2. Rorschach H. [Zur Pathologie und Operabilitat der Zirbeldruse]. Beitr Z Klin Chir 1913;83:451 [in German].
3. Cushing H. Intracranial tumors: notes upon a series of two thousand verified cases with surgical mortality pertaining thereto. Springfield (IL): Charles C. Thomas; 1932.
4. Dandy W. Operative experience in cases of pineal tumor. Arch Surg 1936;33:19–46.
5. van Wagenen WP. A surgical approach for the removal of certain pineal tumors. Surg Gynecol Obstet 1931;37:216–20.
6. Horrax G. Extirpation of a huge pinealoma from a patient with pubertas praecox: a new operative approach. Arch Neurol Psychiatr 1937;37:385–97.
7. Regis J, Bouillot P, Rouby-Volot F, et al. Pineal region tumors and the role of stereotactic biopsy: review of the mortality, morbidity, and diagnostic rates in 370 cases. Neurosurgery 1996;39(5):907–12 [discussion: 912–4].
8. Stein BM. The infratentorial supracerebellar approach to pineal lesions. J Neurosurg 1971;35(2):197–202.
9. Jamieson KG. Excision of pineal tumors. J Neurosurg 1971;35(5):550–3.
10. Pecker J, Scarabin JM, Brucher JM, et al. [Contribution of stereotactic methods to diagnosis and treatment of tumors of the pineal region (author's

transl)]. Rev Neurol (Paris) 1978;134(4):287–94 [in French].

11. Backlund EO, Rahn T, Sarby B. Treatment of pinealomas by stereotaxic radiation surgery. Acta Radiol Ther Phys Biol 1974;13(4):368–76.

12. Choi JU, Kim DS, Chung SS, et al. Treatment of germ cell tumors in the pineal region. Childs Nerv Syst 1998;14(1–2):41–8.

13. Bruce J. Pineal tumors. In: Winn H, editor. Youman's neurological surgery. Philadelphia: WB Saunders Company; 2004. p. 1011–29.

14. Goodman RR. Magnetic resonance imaging-directed stereotactic endoscopic third ventriculostomy. Neurosurgery 1993;32(6):1043–7 [discussion: 1047].

15. Bruce JN, Stein BM. Surgical management of pineal region tumors. Acta Neurochir (Wien) 1995;134(3–4):130–5.

16. Dempsey PK, Kondziolka D, Lunsford LD. Stereotactic diagnosis and treatment of pineal region tumours and vascular malformations. Acta Neurochir (Wien) 1992;116(1):14–22.

17. Edwards MS, Hudgins RJ, Wilson CB, et al. Pineal region tumors in children. J Neurosurg 1988;68(5):689–97.

18. Fauchon F, Jouvet A, Paquis P, et al. Parenchymal pineal tumors: a clinicopathological study of 76 cases. Int J Radiat Oncol Biol Phys 2000;46(4):959–68.

19. Konovalov AN, Pitskhelauri DI. Principles of treatment of the pineal region tumors. Surg Neurol 2003;59(4):250–68.

20. Lapras C, Patet JD, Mottolese C, et al. Direct surgery for pineal tumors: occipital-transtentorial approach. Prog Exp Tumor Res 1987;30:268–80.

21. Neuwelt EA. An update on the surgical treatment of malignant pineal region tumors. Clin Neurosurg 1985;32:397–428.

22. Pluchino F, Broggi G, Fornari M, et al. Surgical approach to pineal tumours. Acta Neurochir (Wien) 1989;96(1–2):26–31.

23. Stein BM. Supracerebellar-infratentorial approach to pineal tumors. Surg Neurol 1979;11(5):331–7.

24. Stein BM, Bruce JN. Surgical management of pineal region tumors (honored guest lecture). Clin Neurosurg 1992;39:509–32.

25. Kraichoke S, Cosgrove M, Chandrasoma PT. Granulomatous inflammation in pineal germinoma. A cause of diagnostic failure at stereotaxic brain biopsy. Am J Surg Pathol 1988;12(9):655–60.

26. Barnett DW, Olson JJ, Thomas WG, et al. Low-grade astrocytomas arising from the pineal gland. Surg Neurol 1995;43(1):70–5 [discussion: 75–6].

27. MacKay CI, Baeesa SS, Ventureyra EC. Epidermoid cysts of the pineal region. Childs Nerv Syst 1999;15(4):170–8.

28. Vaquero J, Ramiro J, Martinez R, et al. Clinicopathological experience with pineocytomas: report of five surgically treated cases. Neurosurgery 1990;27(4):612–8 [discussion: 618–9].

29. Lutterbach J, Fauchon F, Schild SE, et al. Malignant pineal parenchymal tumors in adult patients: patterns of care and prognostic factors. Neurosurgery 2002;51(1):44–55 [discussion: 55–6].

30. Matsutani M, Sano K, Takakura K, et al. Primary intracranial germ cell tumors: a clinical analysis of 153 histologically verified cases. J Neurosurg 1997;86(3):446–55.

31. Mena H, Rushing EJ, Ribas JL, et al. Tumors of pineal parenchymal cells: a correlation of histological features, including nucleolar organizer regions, with survival in 35 cases. Hum Pathol 1995;26(1):20–30.

32. Reddy AT, Janss AJ, Phillips PC, et al. Outcome for children with supratentorial primitive neuroectodermal tumors treated with surgery, radiation, and chemotherapy. Cancer 2000;88(9):2189–93.

33. Schild SE, Scheithauer BW, Haddock MG, et al. Histologically confirmed pineal tumors and other germ cell tumors of the brain. Cancer 1996;78(12):2564–71.

34. Schild SE, Scheithauer BW, Schomberg PJ, et al. Pineal parenchymal tumors. Clinical, pathologic, and therapeutic aspects. Cancer 1993;72(3):870–80.

35. Weiner HL, Finlay JL. Surgery in the management of primary intracranial germ cell tumors. Childs Nerv Syst 1999;15(11–12):770–3.

36. Gaab MR, Schroeder HW. Neuroendoscopic approach to intraventricular lesions. J Neurosurg 1998;88(3):496–505.

37. Pople IK, Athanasiou TC, Sandeman DR, et al. The role of endoscopic biopsy and third ventriculostomy in the management of pineal region tumours. Br J Neurosurg 2001;15(4):305–11.

38. Yamini B, Refai D, Rubin CM, et al. Initial endoscopic management of pineal region tumors and associated hydrocephalus: clinical series and literature review. J Neurosurg 2004;100(5 Suppl Pediatrics):437–41.

39. Ferrer E, Santamarta D, Garcia-Fructuoso G, et al. Neuroendoscopic management of pineal region tumours. Acta Neurochir (Wien) 1997;139(1):12–20 [discussion: 20–1].

40. Chernov MF, Kamikawa S, Yamane F, et al. Neurofiberscopic biopsy of tumors of the pineal region and posterior third ventricle: indications, technique, complications, and results. Neurosurgery 2006;59(2):267–77 [discussion: 267–77].

41. Morgenstern PF, Osbun N, Schwartz TH, et al. Pineal region tumors: an optimal approach for simultaneous endoscopic third ventriculostomy and biopsy. Neurosurg Focus 2011;30(4):E3.

42. Oppido PA, Fiorindi A, Benvenuti L, et al. Neuroendoscopic biopsy of ventricular tumors: a multicentric experience. Neurosurg Focus 2011;30(4):E2.

43. Bruce JN, Ogden AT. Surgical strategies for treating patients with pineal region tumors. J Neurooncol 2004;69(1–3):221–36.

44. Reid WS, Clark WK. Comparison of the infratentorial and transtentorial approaches to the pineal region. Neurosurgery 1978;3(1):1–8.

45. Bruce JN, Stein B. Posterior third ventricular tumors. In: Kaye AH, Black P, editors. Operative neurosurgery, vol. 1. London: Churchill-Livingstone; 2000. p. 769.

46. Bruce JN, Stein B. Supracerebellar approach to pineal region neoplasms. In: Schmidek HH, Sweet W, editors. Operative neurosurgical techniques. 3rd edition. Philadelphia: WB Saunders; 1995. p. 755.

47. Bruce J. Supracerebellar approach to pineal region neoplasms. In: Schmidek H, editor. Operative neurosurgical techniques. 4th edition. Philadelphia: WB Saunders; 2000. p. 908.

48. Bruce JN, Stein B. Complications of surgery for pineal region tumors. In: Post KD, Friedman E, McCormick P, editors. Postoperative complications in intracranial neurosurgery. New York: Thieme; 1993. p. 74.

49. McComb JG, Apuzzo ML. The lateral decubitus position for the surgical approach to pineal location tumors. Concepts Pediatr Neurosurg 1988;8:186.

50. Ausman JI, Malik GM, Dujovny M, et al. Three-quarter prone approach to the pineal-tentorial region. Surg Neurol 1988;29(4):298–306.

51. Ueyama T, Al-Mefty O, Tamaki N. Bridging veins on the tentorial surface of the cerebellum: a microsurgical anatomic study and operative considerations. Neurosurgery 1998;43(5):1137–45.

52. McComb J, Levy ML, Apuzzo M. The posterior intrahemispheric retrocallosal and transcallosal approaches to the third ventricle region. In: Apuzzo M, editor. Surgery of the third ventricle. 2nd edition. Baltimore (MD): Williams & Wilkins; 1998. p. 743.

53. Apuzzo M, Tunk H. Supratentorial approaches to the pineal region. In: Apuzzo M, editor. Brain surgery: complication avoidance and management. New York: Churchill-Livingstone; 1993. p. 486.

54. Bruce J. Management of pineal region tumors. Neurosurg Quart 1993;3:103–19.

55. Chandy MJ, Damaraju SC. Benign tumours of the pineal region: a prospective study from 1983 to 1997. Br J Neurosurg 1998;12(3):228–33.

56. Fetell MR, Bruce JN, Burke AM, et al. Non-neoplastic pineal cysts. Neurology 1991;41(7):1034–40.

57. Wolden SL, Wara WM, Larson DA, et al. Radiation therapy for primary intracranial germ-cell tumors. Int J Radiat Oncol Biol Phys 1995;32(4):943–9.

58. Jenkin RD, Simpson WJ, Keen CW. Pineal and suprasellar germinomas. Results of radiation treatment. J Neurosurg 1978;48(1):99–107.

59. Sawamura Y, de Tribolet N, Ishii N, et al. Management of primary intracranial germinomas: diagnostic surgery or radical resection? J Neurosurg 1997;87(2):262–6.

60. Franzini A, Leocata F, Servello D, et al. Long-term follow-up of germinoma after stereotactic biopsy and brain radiotherapy: a cell kinetics study. J Neurol 1998;245(9):593–7.

61. Rich TA, Cassady JR, Strand RD, et al. Radiation therapy for pineal and suprasellar germ cell tumors. Cancer 1985;55(5):932–40.

62. Oi S. Recent advances and racial differences in therapeutic strategy to the pineal region tumor. Childs Nerv Syst 1998;14(1–2):33–5.

63. Oi S, Matsuzawa K, Choi JU, et al. Identical characteristics of the patient populations with pineal region tumors in Japan and in Korea and therapeutic modalities. Childs Nerv Syst 1998;14(1–2):36–40.

64. Kersh CR, Constable WC, Eisert DR, et al. Primary central nervous system germ cell tumors. Effect of histologic confirmation on radiotherapy. Cancer 1988;61(11):2148–52.

65. Matsutani M, Sano K, Takakura K, et al. Combined treatment with chemotherapy and radiation therapy for intracranial germ cell tumors. Childs Nerv Syst 1998;14(1–2):59–62.

66. Camins MB, Schlesinger EB. Treatment of tumours of the posterior part of the third ventricle and the pineal region: a long term follow-up. Acta Neurochir (Wien) 1978;40(1–2):131–43.

67. Robertson PL, DaRosso RC, Allen JC. Improved prognosis of intracranial non-germinoma germ cell tumors with multimodality therapy. J Neurooncol 1997;32(1):71–80.

68. Balmaceda C, Heller G, Rosenblum M, et al. Chemotherapy without irradiation—a novel approach for newly diagnosed CNS germ cell tumors: results of an international cooperative trial. The First International Central Nervous System Germ Cell Tumor Study. J Clin Oncol 1996;14(11):2908–15.

69. Buckner JC, Peethambaram PP, Smithson WA, et al. Phase II trial of primary chemotherapy followed by reduced-dose radiation for CNS germ cell tumors. J Clin Oncol 1999;17(3):933–40.

70. Kochi M, Itoyama Y, Shiraishi S, et al. Successful treatment of intracranial nongerminomatous malignant germ cell tumors by administering neoadjuvant chemotherapy and radiotherapy before excision of residual tumors. J Neurosurg 2003;99(1):106–14.

71. Weiner HL, Lichtenbaum RA, Wisoff JH, et al. Delayed surgical resection of central nervous system germ cell tumors. Neurosurgery 2002;50(4):727–33 [discussion: 733–4].

72. Friedman JA, Lynch JJ, Buckner JC, et al. Management of malignant pineal germ cell tumors with

residual mature teratoma. Neurosurgery 2001;48(3): 518–22 [discussion: 522–3].

73. Jouvet A, Saint-Pierre G, Fauchon F, et al. Pineal parenchymal tumors: a correlation of histological features with prognosis in 66 cases. Brain Pathol 2000;10(1):49–60.

74. Borit A, Blackwood W, Mair WG. The separation of pineocytoma from pineoblastoma. Cancer 1980; 45(6):1408–18.

75. Packer RJ, Sutton LN, Rorke LB, et al. Prognostic importance of cellular differentiation in medullo-blastoma of childhood. J Neurosurg 1984;61(2): 296–301.

76. Graham ML, Herndon JE 2nd, Casey JR, et al. High-dose chemotherapy with autologous stem-cell rescue in patients with recurrent and high-risk pedi-atric brain tumors. J Clin Oncol 1997;15(5):1814–23.

77. Gururangan S, McLaughlin C, Quinn J, et al. High-dose chemotherapy with autologous stem-cell rescue in children and adults with newly diagnosed pineoblastomas. J Clin Oncol 2003;21(11):2187–91.

78. Jakacki RI, Zeltzer PM, Boyett JM, et al. Survival and prognostic factors following radiation and/or chemo-therapy for primitive neuroectodermal tumors of the pineal region in infants and children: a report of the Childrens Cancer Group. J Clin Oncol 1995; 13(6):1377–83.

79. Duffner PK, Cohen ME, Sanford RA, et al. Lack of effi-cacy of postoperative chemotherapy and delayed radiation in very young children with pineoblastoma. Pediatric Oncology Group. Med Pediatr Oncol 1995; 25(1):38–44.

80. Yeh DD, Warnick RE, Ernst RJ. Management strategy for adult patients with dorsal midbrain gliomas. Neurosurgery 2002;50(4):735–8 [discus-sion: 738–40].

81. Hoffman HJ, Yoshida M, Becker LE, et al. Pineal region tumors in childhood. Experience at the hospital for sick children. 1983. Pediatr Neurosurg 1994;21(1):91–103 [discussion: 104].

82. Luo SQ, Li DZ, Zhang MZ, et al. Occipital transen-torial approach for removal of pineal region tumors: report of 64 consecutive cases. Surg Neurol 1989; 32(1):36–9.

83. Herrmann HD, Winkler D, Westphal M. Treatment of tumours of the pineal region and posterior part of the third ventricle. Acta Neurochir (Wien) 1992;116(2–4): 137–46.

84. Kang JK, Jeun SS, Hong YK, et al. Experience with pineal region tumors. Childs Nerv Syst 1998;14(1–2): 63–8.

85. Shin HJ, Cho BK, Jung HW, et al. Pediatric pineal tumors: need for a direct surgical approach and complications of the occipital transtentorial approach. Childs Nerv Syst 1998;14(4–5):174–8.

86. Jia W. Transcallosal interforniceal approach to pineal region tumors in 150 children. J Neurosurg Pediatr 2011;7(1):98–103.

Minimally Invasive Approaches to the Pineal Region

Michael E. Sughrue, MD

KEYWORDS

• Pineal • Minimally invasive • Approach

The pineal-tectal region is an anatomically challenging region to operate in safely. Deeply situated in the brain, it is bounded by and guarded by several critical structures, namely the galenic venous system, the superior cerebellar artery, the 4th nerve, the thalamus, and the midbrain. The tentorium is sharply upsloping and the tentorial cerebellar surface is conformal to this slope, with the apex of the vermis, the culmen, tightly fitting in the apical tentorial cleft, and blocking simple access to the pineal region through a direct approach. It was only through adoption of the operating microscope and the sitting position that the infratentorial-supracerebellar approach to the pineal region began to be widely used to directly attack pineal tumors with good outcomes and minimal morbidity.[1,2]

The present review assesses possible strategies on how to make this significant advance, refined over decades, better, ie, less invasive, while still respecting this delicate region, and achieving anatomic and oncologic goals. Experience with keyhole approaches to this region is somewhat limited in anyone's hands, because there simply are not that many pineal tumors in anyone's practice to gain extensive experience with keyhole pineal surgery. However, an explication of anatomic principles of this region and some basic surgical principles of keyhole surgery are provided to further assist those interested in minimizing surgical impact during pineal surgery. Although this review, for the sake of brevity, focuses on the infratentorial-supracerebellar approach, many of these principles can be adapted to other approaches, such as the occipital transtentorial, without excessive imagination.

KEYHOLE SURGERY

The term keyhole surgery does not refer to a specific technique but to a philosophy that emphasizes using the smallest opening necessary to achieve the anatomic goals of surgery.[3,4] Although it is difficult to prove that smaller craniotomies are better than larger ones, larger craniotomies expose more brain surface to the air and microscope light (ie, nonphysiologic conditions) for longer periods of time, and larger incisions are generally more prone to wound complications and pain than smaller ones.[3,4] However, this does not imply that it is wise to make the opening so small that dangerous maneuvers, or lack of visualization, are part of the surgery; in some cases keyhole craniotomies might be large. Instead, it implies that the least exposure necessary is the optimal exposure.

Keyhole surgery requires some modification of traditional techniques.[5] Most notably, the smaller hole requires more frequent alterations of the viewing angle to achieve all the necessary views.[3,5] The patient should be secured to the bed in all directions to ensure safety with frequent repositioning, and the surgeon should be prepared to frequently adjust the microscope.[3,5] A mouthpiece adjustment device might be helpful for this. In addition, endoscope assistance might be necessary to achieve otherwise challenging angles of visualization. Using a keyhole approach requires a degree of planning not needed with larger conventional craniotomies, because it is much harder to adjust the approach midsurgery. Image guidance is essential, and obtaining accurate registration is more important in these cases

Comprehensive Brain Tumor Center, Department of Neurological Surgery, University of Oklahoma, 1000 North Lincoln Boulevard, Suite 400, Oklahoma City, OK 73104-5023, USA
E-mail address: mes261@columbia.edu

Neurosurg Clin N Am 22 (2011) 381–384
doi:10.1016/j.nec.2011.05.005
1042-3680/11/$ – see front matter © 2011 Elsevier Inc. All rights reserved.

generally, because you do not always get all the angles of visualization you might in a larger craniotomy. Keyhole surgery requires patience in a way that is not always seen with larger craniotomies.[6] Although the work required to do a smaller exposure is less, each step requires more attention to detail and a conscious effort to slow down, because minor imperfections are less tolerated in a small space, and the time needed to drain more cerebrospinal fluid and get the brain out of the way before beginning arachnoidal dissection and intradural work is longer.

WHY KEYHOLE SURGERY FOR THE PINEAL REGION?

Although the thought of working in a small hole deep in the head is unnerving to some experienced in this surgery, there are a lot of reasons to think that openings can be made smaller in keyhole surgeries. First, although it might be comforting to have a lot of exposure, it is likely that most people do not use the entire craniotomy for performing this approach. Although the tentorium is a broad structure, the aperture at the apex when approaching from posteriorly is narrow (**Fig. 1**), and ultimately this limits the working space at the target region far more than the size of the craniotomy. Most pathologic lesions in this region are midline and generally do not require extremely wide working angles. Careful planning can select tumors for which significant off-midline working angles are needed and tailor the craniotomies to these cases appropriately. There is no need to expose the entire cerebellar hemisphere (potentially injuring it in the process) when access to the superior surface is all that is needed.[3] Exposing

down to the foramen magnum in the supracerebellar approach does not obviate the need for gentle downward retraction of the cerebellar culmen in these cases, however it does increase the amount of muscle and soft tissue dissection, which is a key source of postoperative pain and wound complications.

Endoscopic assistance can be a significant help in keyhole surgery. Typically, one of the greatest dangers with the use of the endoscope is the danger to critical structures in the endoscope's blind spot, which can be injured when the endoscope strikes these structures during movement or resting.[6] The pineal region is uniquely privileged in this respect, because the trajectory between the dura and the target is largely free of critical structures following sacrifice of the bridging veins and padding of the cerebellum (see **Fig. 1**). Thus, the pineal region is an ideal location for the use of endoscopic assistance, which can be of great help when visualizing a laterally located tumor and anatomy underneath the tentorial edge.

KEYHOLE SURGERY FOR THE PINEAL REGION
Planning

Keyhole surgery requires more planning than the typical surgical approach, because it is less robust to mistakes than other approaches. First, the center of the lesion should be defined as specifically as possible given the extent of the lesion, and the edges of the mass should be defined in terms of this centroid. By thinking of the tumor in this fashion, one can best assess the overall appropriateness of a given approach, such as the infratentorial-supracerebellar approach; it is better to have the periphery of the tumor just

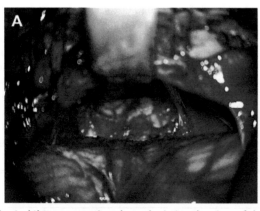 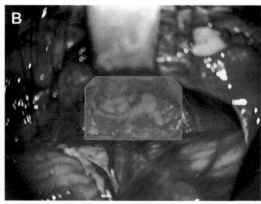

Fig. 1. (*A*) Intraoperative photo depicting the view of the pineal region and posterior tentorial incisura following a pineal tumor resection in the sitting position via a conventional craniotomy. This picture nicely demonstrates the significant amount of bone work performed in traditional approaches that can potentially be omitted because it does not permit useful working angles. (*B*) The same image with the effective working space of the pineal region shaded in blue.

outside the angles of easy accessibility than the central bulk of the tumor. Also by getting a sense of how far this tumor is tucked beneath the tentorial insura at the falcotentorial junction, and the angle of the tentorial slope, the relative merits of the sitting versus prone positioning can be appreciated. The position of the galenic venous system, including the internal cerebral veins, relative to the tumor should be noted. This position is best noted on the T2 images in many cases.

The anticipated pathologic lesion is also important to be taken into consideration. Pineal parenchymal tumors should undergo gross total removal if at all possible, and the approach selection should provide every opportunity to ensure that this happens first and foremost.[7,8] Other tumors, such as low-lying falcotentorial meningiomas, can be subtotally resected, if necessary, with good long-term results with observation or radiosurgical treatment of the remnant.[9] Other cases, such as germ cell neoplasms or exophytic low-grade gliomas, are usually only biopsied, which makes these lesions ideal for minimally invasive techniques. Thus, although a giant pineoblastoma tucked under a high sloping tentorium might necessitate a full cerebellar exposure, this extra work might be avoided in a smaller more localized tumor.

Positioning

Whenever possible (namely the absence of a patent foramen ovale), the sitting approach provides the best exposure to the pineal region for several reasons. The cerebellum is more relaxed by the lower venous tension, and the working corridor is generally excellent. The logistical challenges of climbing the tentorial surface in the prone position are less discussed. Microsurgery is generally better performed sitting comfortably, however it is difficult in the author's experience to work backward in this angle while sitting with the patient prone and the surgeon at the patients head. Standing surgery on the pineal gland makes it easier to see this angle, however is less comfortable and less ergonomic than sitting. Operating with the patient in the sitting position raises its own ergonomic challenges, however by appropriately positioning the surgical armrest and leaning the patient forward, a flat and reasonably comfortable surgical trajectory can be obtained.

As with all keyhole surgery, minor positioning errors are less tolerated than with larger openings. The head should ideally be midline, not laterally flexed, with slight rotation away from a specific side if lateral extension under the tentorium is present. Forward flexion should be maximized, however evoked potentials before and after positioning should confirm the absence of overflexion.

The potentials generally become useless during the surgery when air accumulates under the calvarium.

Exposure

The target bone flap is centered around the inion exposing the torcula and adjacent portions of the sinuses completely so that the torcula can be gently retracted superiorly to improve exposure (see **Fig. 1**A). The lateral extension is a few centimeters lateral to inion and should be tailored to each case. It is probably helpful to cheat the bone flap larger toward the side of the surgeon's dominant hand to increase the available working angles. In contrast to a more traditional suboccipital exposure, the bone flap need only extend downwards approximately 2 to 3 cm below the torcula (**Fig. 2**), and it is only necessary to dissect slightly more suboccipital musculature than that, given that this is a frequent cause of postoperative pain. Image guidance is obviously invaluable in defining these sinus boundaries.

The decision to perform craniotomy versus craniectomy is individualized based on age, however it is usually possible to raise a bone flap in most cases without a problem if 4 burr holes are made around the torcula and the dura over the sinuses is stripped before turning the craniotomy.

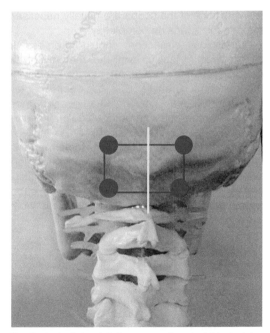

Fig. 2. A skull model demonstrating the skin incision (approx 5 cm, does not extend below the foramen magnum) in yellow and the bone flap and burr holes (approx 3.5 cm each edge) in red. This flap can and should be modified to specific cases as needed.

Although the risk of venous air embolus should force one to err on the side of not risking a sinus tear, the dura typically strips easily in the sitting position if done carefully, and replacing a bone flap makes repair easier and reduces the risk of complications compared with mesh alone.

The dura is opened in the traditional V shape, however given the broader base to length ratio in these shorter flaps, it is probably useful to make the base narrower than typical, given the importance of being able to retract and fold the dura and torcula upward in these cases.

Intradural Work

Although the lack of cerebellar sag that occurs in a smaller craniotomy makes dural closure easier, it does make the working window smaller initially than many are used to. Like all keyhole surgery, patience and thorough arachnoidal dissection is critical to safe surgery. All superior bridging cerebellar veins should be sacrificed (see **Fig. 1**A) and the thick arachnoid should be dissected on both sides from lateral to medial approaching the midline arachnoid. The use of 2 retractor blades, one to gently elevate the torcula and the other to slightly depress the cerebellar vermis, may be needed at this stage, however the cerebellum is usually softer and more tolerant of this retraction than when prone, especially when padded with pieces of rubber glove and cottonoids. Multiple reangulations of the scope are usually necessary to open this space up completely.

Arachnoidal dissection should progress in a goal-directed fashion until the anatomy of the galenic system is obvious. After clearly identifying the precentral cerebellar vein, this vein is cauterized and divided. The eventual goal in most surgeries is to place a retractor blade on the anterior portion of the cerebellar culmen to facilitate visualization of the pineal and tectal regions. Once this has been accomplished, surgery progresses as dictated by the pathoanatomy. Difficult angles of view can be achieved with an endoscope, which can be introduced with less worry

of injury to more superficial structures, which should be well padded. The inherent problems with the introduction of a 30° endoscope are less problematic in this region, and the 30° is able to provide some visualization of difficult regions of lateral anatomy not possible with a microscope.

Closure

Closure is typically simpler than with a traditional suboccipital approach, especially given that the cerebellum is not protruding into the lower extent of the dural opening as it would if the occipital squamosa were removed.

REFERENCES

1. Pople IK, Athanasiou TC, Sandeman DR, et al. The role of endoscopic biopsy and third ventriculostomy in the management of pineal region tumours. Br J Neurosurg 2001;15(4):305–11.
2. Portillo ML, de Gonzalez CM, Sangines JB, et al. Pineal region tumors. Int Surg 1982;67(4):329–33.
3. Perneczy A, Reisch R. Keyhole approaches in neurosurgery. New York: Springer Wien; 2008.
4. Sughrue ME, Teo C. Neurosurgery Clinics of North America. Minimally invasive intracranial surgery [Preface]. Neurosurg Clin N Am 2010;21(4):xi.
5. Teo C. The concept of minimally invasive neurosurgery. Neurosurg Clin N Am 2010;21(4):583–4, v.
6. Sughrue ME, Mills SA, Young RL 2nd. Complication avoidance in minimally invasive neurosurgery. Neurosurg Clin N Am 2010;21(4):699–702, vii–viii.
7. Clark AJ, Sughrue ME, Ivan ME, et al. Factors influencing overall survival rates for patients with pineocytoma. J Neurooncol 2010;100(2):255–60.
8. Clark AJ, Ivan ME, Sughrue ME, et al. Tumor control after surgery and radiotherapy for pineocytoma. J Neurosurg 2010;113(2):319–24.
9. Sughrue ME, Kane AJ, Shangari G, et al. The relevance of Simpson Grade I and II resection in modern neurosurgical treatment of World Health Organization Grade I meningiomas. J Neurosurg 2010;113(5):1029–35.

Clinical Outcomes after Treatment of Germ Cell Tumors

Christopher Jackson, BA[a,b], George Jallo, MD[a,b],
Michael Lim, MD[a,b],*

KEYWORDS

- Germ cell tumors • Germinomas
- Nongerminomatous germ cell tumors • Intracranial GCTs

Germ cell tumors (GCTs) are neoplasms of gonadal origin and are broadly classified as germinomas, nongerminomatous germ cell tumors (NGGCTs), or mixed tumors.[1] Germinomas arise from primordial germ cells, whereas NGGCTs (teratoma, embryonal carcinoma, endodermal sinus tumor, and choriocarcinoma) arise from cells of the differentiated embryo, undifferentiated embryo, yolk sac endoderm, and trophoblast, respectively.[2,3] With the exception of mature teratomas, GCTs are uniformly malignant. Among pure tumors, germinomas are the least aggressive, followed by immature teratomas, embryonal carcinomas, and choriocarcinomas.[4] For mixed tumors, aggressiveness is determined by the proportion of the tumor mass contributed by each cell type.[4,5] GCTs can be further classified as secreting or nonsecreting. Secreting tumors are characterized by elevation of alpha-fetoprotein (AFP) and/or beta-human chorionic gonadotropin (beta-hCG) in the cerebrospinal fluid (CSF) and/or serum. Although there is considerable variability in expression of AFP and beta-hCG among GCTs, secreting tumors are generally considered more aggressive than their nonsecreting counterparts.[6–8] One notable exception is a subset of germinomas that contain syncytiotrophoblasts, which secrete low levels of beta-hCG, but clinically behave like pure germinomas.[9]

GCTs typically arise in the gonads; however, 2% to 3% of primary GCTs are extragonadal.[3]

Because of the pattern of migration of primitive germ cells during embryonic development, extragonadal GCTs characteristically form in midline structures within the retroperitoneum, anterior mediastinum, and central nervous system (CNS).[10,11] In the CNS, GCTs exhibit the same midline pattern of distribution observed in other body sites, with most tumors developing in the pineal region (56%) or suprasellar compartment (28%).[3,12] Less frequent sites of primary intracranial GCTs include the basal ganglia, thalamus, cerebellum, lateral ventricle, cerebellopontine angle, corpus callosum, and spinal cord.[13] GCTs may also be bifocal in 6% to 41% of cases and are most frequently observed simultaneously in the pineal and suprasellar regions.[14,15] Approximately 65% of intracranial GCTs are classified as germinomas, 18% are teratomas, 5% are embryonal carcinomas, 7% are endodermal sinus tumors, and 5% are choriocarcinomas.[16] In practice, only teratoma and germinoma are frequently encountered as pure neoplasms and approximately 25% of all GCTs are mixed tumors.[4,17]

GCTs account for 0.3% to 3.4% of all intracranial tumors in Western countries; however, they are considerably more common in Asian countries and represent 4.8% to 15.0% of pediatric brain tumors in Japan.[3,5,18,19] GCTs are typically diagnosed in pediatric or adolescent patients with the peak incidence of intracranial GCTs early in the second decade of life.[3,16] Males are at an

[a] Department of Neurosurgery, The Johns Hopkins University School of Medicine, Phipps 123, 600 North Wolfe Street, Baltimore, MD 21287, USA
[b] Department of Oncology, The Johns Hopkins University School of Medicine, Phipps 123, 600 North Wolfe Street, Baltimore, MD 21287, USA
* Corresponding author. Department of Neurosurgery, The Johns Hopkins University School of Medicine, Phipps 123, 600 North Wolfe Street, Baltimore, MD 21287.
E-mail address: mlim3@jhmi.edu

Neurosurg Clin N Am 22 (2011) 385–394
doi:10.1016/j.nec.2011.04.002
1042-3680/11/$ – see front matter © 2011 Elsevier Inc. All rights reserved.

increased risk of developing intracranial GCTs with a male-to-female ratio reported between 1.5:1.0 and 3.0:1.0.[5,20] An increased incidence of both intracranial and extracranial GCTs has also been reported in patients with certain chromosomal disorders, including Klinefelter syndrome and Down syndrome.[21,22] Although the incidence of intracranial GCTs remains relatively low, the proportion of intracranial tumors represented by GCTs has been gradually, but steadily increasing worldwide.[21] This observation, taken with the well-documented geographic distribution of these tumors and the observed association with chromosomal abnormalities, lends support to the hypothesis that environmental and genetic factors likely play a role in the pathogenesis of this diverse group of neoplasms.[23,24]

The presenting signs and symptoms of intracranial GCTs vary with tumor location. Pineal tumors frequently occlude the cerebral aqueduct and patients present with signs and symptoms of elevated intracranial pressure secondary to hydrocephalus.[16] When the tumor compresses the midbrain, patients frequently present with oculomotor abnormalities, including pupils that react better to accommodation than light, lid retraction, convergence abnormalities, and failure of upward gaze (Parinaud syndrome).[16,25] Suprasellar tumors commonly present with hypothalamic/pituitary axis dysfunction, including diabetes insipidis, delayed or precocious puberty, adrenal insufficiency, or symptoms of growth hormone deficiency.[25,26]

Although intracranial GCTs can be readily detected with computed tomography (CT), magnetic resonance imaging (MRI) remains the imaging modality of choice for detecting, characterizing, and staging these tumors (**Fig. 1**). GCTs are generally isointense or low signal intensity on T1-weighted images and isointense or high signal intensity on T2-weighted images.[16] It has been suggested that certain GCT subtypes may have characteristic MRI signals[27,28]; however, MRI alone has not been shown to be adequately sensitive or specific to obviate the need for histologic diagnosis.[28,29] If a GCT is suspected, MRI of the spine is a critical step in staging, as spinal cord involvement is present in up to 10% of patients at the time of diagnosis.[2] CSF cytology should also be obtained for staging, as patients with positive CSF cytology are considered to have metastatic disease even in the absence of MRI findings.[30] Hematogenous spread to extraneural sites at the time of diagnosis has also been described,[31] but this is an exceedingly rare occurrence.

Measurement of CSF and serum beta-hCG and AFP may also aid in diagnosis and some investigators have suggested that significant elevation of these markers in the setting of imaging findings suggestive of aggressive disease may justify forgoing biopsy in favor of prompt treatment with radiotherapy and chemotherapy.[8] Similarly, imaging findings suggestive of pure germinoma in the absence of positive tumor markers may justify forgoing histologic diagnosis to begin radiotherapy immediately.[27] This approach, however, remains controversial. Unless tumor markers and radiology unequivocally indicate a specific diagnosis, the consensus is that tissue should be obtained for histologic evaluation in all patients who are able to tolerate the procedure. The preferred method for obtaining tissue is also controversial. Some investigators have suggested that open biopsy may facilitate more accurate diagnosis.[32,33] Others maintain that stereotactic biopsy interpreted in the context of serum and CSF tumor markers is preferred to avoid the inherent risks of surgery in the pineal and suprasellar regions.[32,34] With either approach, discordance between histology and tumor markers likely represents a mixed tumor and should be treated as the more aggressive subtype.

TREATMENT APPROACHES AND CLINICAL OUTCOMES

Identifying the optimal treatment approach for primary intracranial GCTs remains a topic of active research in the field of neuro-oncology. Because of the diversity of this rare group of neoplasms, there is a paucity of well-controlled prospective trials. Available data from retrospective studies is often difficult to interpret, as these studies tend to be relatively small and heterogeneous. An algorithm for the diagnosis and treatment of GCTs is depicted in **Fig. 2**. Here we review the management of intracranial GCTs and discuss the clinical outcomes of patients who undergo treatment for these rare and fascinating tumors.

Germinomas

Germinomas are extraordinarily radiosensitive, and 5-year to 10-year survival rates in excess of 90% have been consistently reported with radiotherapy alone.[13,29,35–38] Given the high success rate of established treatment regimens at controlling local and distant disease progression, the focus has more recently shifted to minimizing late radiation effects in this generally young patient population.[18,33,35,39] Historically, the standard of care has been 45 to 55 Gy administered to the primary tumor site with 30 to 36 Gy to the entire craniospinal axis to reduce the risk of leptomeningeal spread.[3,16,39–41] However, with 20-year survival rates in excess of 80% reported in some series,[13] even relatively low doses of radiation

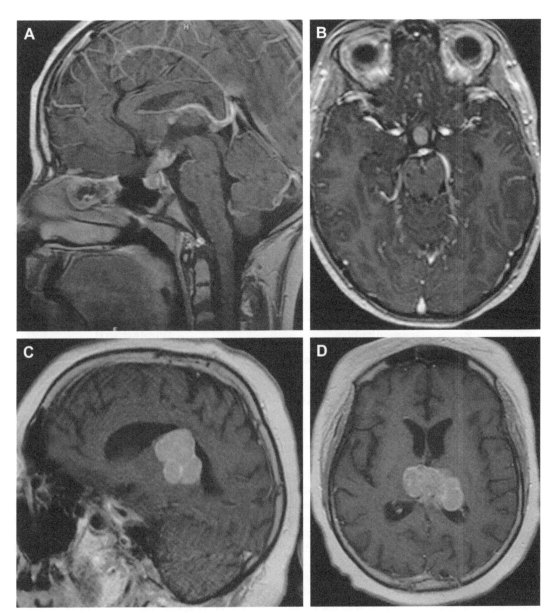

Fig. 1. Contrast-enhanced T1-weighted MRI images of a germinoma involving the infundibular stalk in an 11-year-old male in sagittal (*A*) and axial (*B*) planes. Contrast-enhanced T1-weighted MRI images of a recurrent NGGCT in an 18-year-old female in sagittal (*C*) and axial (*D*) planes.

raise concern for long-term sequelae. Neurocognitive dysfunction has been well-documented in patients receiving as little as 20 to 25 Gy for treatment of brain tumors.[42] Adverse physical effects of radiotherapy have also been reported, including hypothalamic-pituitary dysfunction, radiation-induced occlusive vasculopathy of large intracranial arteries, an increased estimated stroke rate (11.7%, 16 years after treatment), development of arteriovenous malformations, and a high estimated rate of secondary neoplasms (16.8%, 19 years after treatment).[43] Broad quality-of-life measures, such as marriage, graduation from high school, and employment, are also negatively impacted by exposure to radiotherapy at a young age.[44] In addition, a study examining the self-reported physical and psychological well-being of patients treated for intracranial germinomas reported a direct correlation between poor functional status and early age of diagnosis.[45] These findings suggest that

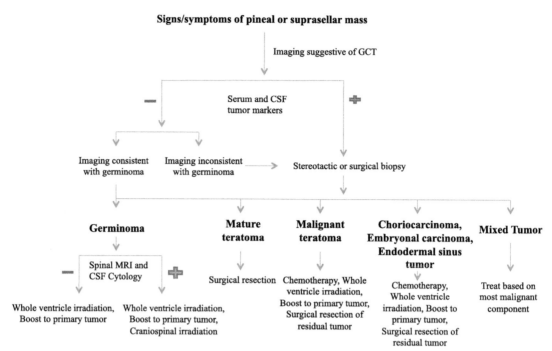

Fig. 2. Algorithm for the diagnosis and treatment of intracranial GCTs.

young patients may be especially vulnerable to the late effects of radiotherapy.

A variety of protocols have been designed to decrease radiation exposure in patients being treated for intracranial germinomas. Common strategies include chemotherapy, stereotactic radiosurgery, dose reduction, field reduction, volume-based dose selection, or a combination of these approaches.[1,12,18,39–41,46–49] Although some investigators have reported improved control of intracranial and spinal disease with radiation doses in excess of 40 Gy and upfront craniospinal radiation,[49–51] this effect has not been consistently demonstrated. Therefore, the current standard of care at most institutions is 21 to 24 Gy to the whole ventricle and an additional boost of 40 to 45 Gy to the primary tumor with craniospinal irradiation reserved for patients with evidence of disseminated disease based on imaging or CSF histology.[16,37,48] Chemotherapy may be added to this regimen for patients with extensive or recurrent disease.[16] Regardless of the initial treatment regimen, patients who achieve complete tumor remission rarely experience recurrence. When tumors do recur, they may be highly aggressive[52]; however, salvage radiotherapy with or without chemotherapy induces lasting remission in the vast majority of cases.[13,53,54]

A limited number of trials have evaluated the effectiveness of stereotactic radiosurgery in the treatment of intracranial germinomas. A case

report by Regine and colleagues,[55] which describes a patient who underwent radiosurgery and refused further treatment, reported no disease recurrence at 6 months. This case highlights the potential of radiosurgery for controlling the primary lesion; however, a combined approach with 10 to 12 Gy delivered to the primary lesion with stereotactic radiosurgery plus whole-ventricular irradiation (24 Gy) is preferred to reduce the risk of leptomeningeal spread as well as interventricular recurrence.[47] This protocol has been reported to provide control rates comparable to traditional radiotherapy regimens.[47,56] It has also been suggested that stereotactic radiosurgery may reduce length of hospital stay and overall treatment costs.[47] Additional studies are warranted to evaluate the effectiveness and economic impact of stereotactic radiosurgery in these patients.

Trials of chemotherapy alone have consistently reported lower rates of remission as compared with radiotherapy or a combination of radiotherapy and chemotherapy.[53,57] Chemotherapy-only regimens have been demonstrated to induce remission at rates in excess of 80%[6]; however, these effects are transient and recurrence rates in the range of 50% have been consistently reported.[6,53,57] A recent international study reported that 7 of 11 patients treated with 4 to 6 cycles of carboplatin/ etoposide alternating with cyclophosphamide/ etoposide relapsed between 13 months and 5 years after diagnosis.[53] This study represented the third of 3 consecutive international cohort studies evaluating a chemotherapy-only approach for intracranial GCTs. Based on the cumulative results of these trials, the investigators concluded that chemotherapy alone offered unacceptably low rates of durable tumor control as compared with either radiotherapy alone or in combination with chemotherapy.[53,57]

Although chemotherapy alone offers inferior tumor control rates compared with radiotherapy, several investigators have reported that neoadjuvant chemotherapy may reduce the dose of radiation required to induce lasting remission.[1,12,46,58] Available data indicate that the addition of chemotherapy allows for a slight dose reduction in whole-ventricle irradiation (21.6–25.5 Gy) and a larger reduction in primary site boost (30.0–30.6 Gy) without compromising tumor control rates.[1,12,46] Severe chemotherapy-related toxicities reported in these studies have primarily been related to myelosuppression. One study of 17 patients treated with etoposide and cisplatin reported neutropenia requiring administration of granulocyte-colony stimulating factor in 5 patients with leukocyte nadirs below 1000/μL in 3 patients. Thrombocytopenia requiring platelet transfusions was reported in 3 patients and 1 patient dropped below 20,000/μL.[46] Nonhematologic toxicities included mild ototoxicity, vomiting, renal insufficiency, and neuropathy. Other studies reported similar rates of adverse events with reported toxicities specific to the chosen chemotherapeutic regimen. Although available data indicate that the radiation doses used in these trials may reduce the rate of early neurocognitive sequelae,[12] to date there is inadequate follow-up to draw meaningful conclusions regarding the late neurocognitive effects of these regimens. Given the established efficacy of whole-ventricle radiotherapy and local radiation boost with the addition of craniospinal radiation for extensive disease, combination approaches of chemotherapy and reduced radiation doses should likely remain restricted to experimental protocols at this time. In the setting of recurrent or extensive disease, however, the addition of chemotherapy to a standard radiotherapy regimen has been shown to improve remission rates.[16] Chemotherapy may also be indicated in patients with a ventriculoperitoneal shunt to decrease the risk of extraneural metastases.[54,59,60]

Given the radiosensitivity of pure germinomas and the risk of surgery in the pineal and suprasellar regions, the role of surgical resection in the treatment of this disease has historically been limited. Advances in microsurgery and endoscopic neurosurgery, however, have led to a reexamination of the role of surgery in the management of these tumors. Although stereotactic biopsy can be prone to diagnostic inaccuracy, endoscopic biopsy has been reported to offer diagnostic yields as high as 90% to 98%.[33] Endoscopic surgery may also afford more accurate assessment of ventricular tumor extension than MRI alone. Given the documented cases of extraneural spread from VP shunts, there has been some concern regarding iatrogenic seeding of endoscopic tracts. Although additional studies are needed to evaluate this potential risk more thoroughly, early reports indicate that rates of tumor dissemination are not increased with endoscopic surgery.[33]

Although extensive resection of germinomas is not currently standard of care, some investigators suggest that the increased diagnostic accuracy afforded by generous tumor sampling should be reevaluated in light of the reduced operative risks associated with modern endoscopic and microsurgical techniques.[32,33] Furthermore, studies of chemotherapy-only therapy for intracranial germinomas have demonstrated a reduction in recurrence for smaller tumors as compared with larger tumors.[57] Although the rate of recurrence is still higher than that observed in radiation protocols, these findings suggest that there may be a future role for cytoreductive surgery with or without chemotherapy, as the field continues to move toward minimizing radiation exposure in these patients.[57]

Nongerminomatous Germ Cell Tumors

NGGCTs are a heterogeneous group of neoplasms that are less common than germinomas and, as a result, available data are sparse and somewhat difficult to interpret. Unlike germinomas, NGGCTs are relatively insensitive to radiotherapy and carry a graver prognosis.[2] Patients treated with a regimen of whole-ventricle irradiation and boost to the lesion have 5-year survival rates in the range of 35% to 60%.[2,13,18,19,61] Nevertheless, radiotherapy remains a critical component of treatment for NGGCTs, as chemotherapy-only regimens have been reported to offer only slightly improved 2-year survival over radiotherapy alone and comparable 5-year survival rates.[6,53] Combination regimens of chemotherapy plus radiotherapy offer improved overall survival with 5-year survival rates consistently reported in the range of 50% to 70%[7,13,34] and higher rates reported in some smaller series.[46,62] Importantly, in a series of 153 histologically confirmed intracranial germ cell tumors (90 NGGCTs), Matsutani and colleagues[13] reported that survival varied significantly based on the histologic subtype of NGGCT. Patients with pure endodermal sinus tumors, choriocarcinomas, or embryonal carcinomas had a 3-year

Table 1
Summary of common treatment approaches and associated outcomes for intracranial germ cell tumors

Tumor Type	PFS	Side Effects and Other Considerations
High-dose Radiotherapy		
Germinoma	>90% at 10 years	High-dose radiotherapy is associated with an increased
Mature teratoma	—	incidence of late neurocognitive effects, endocrine
Other NGGCT	35%–60% at 5 years	dysfunction, cerebrovascular disease, secondary neoplasms, and decreased quality of life based on subjective well-being, as well as objective measures such as marriage rate, graduation from high school, employment, and successful completion of college.
Reduced-dose Radiotherapy		
Germinoma	>90% at 10 years	Reduced-dose radiotherapy has been shown to offer
Mature teratoma	—	comparable disease control rates as high-dose
Other NGGCT	—	radiotherapy for germinoma. This approach has the theoretical benefit of decreased late radiation effects.
Chemotherapy		
Germinoma	50% at 3 years	Chemotherapy alone has consistently been shown to be
Mature teratoma	—	inferior to radiotherapy.
Other NGGCT	35%–50% at 5 years	
Chemotherapy with High-dose Radiotherapy		
Germinoma	—	This is the treatment of choice for malignant NGGCTs. Long-
Mature teratoma	—	term survivors likely suffer from late radiation effects, but
Other NGGCT	50%–70% at 5 years	the threat of mortality posed by these tumors is currently felt to justify this approach.
Chemotherapy with Reduced-dose Radiotherapy		
Germinoma	>90% at 10 years	Although recurrence of pure germinomas is rare, this
Mature Teratoma	—	treatment approach offers a high rate of second remission.
Other NGGCT	35% at 5 years	Neoadjuvant chemotherapy with reduced-dose radiotherapy is also the treatment of choice for patients with disseminated disease at the time of diagnosis as well as for patients with VP shunts. The PFS rate reported here for NGGCTs is based on only 2 small studies and should be interpreted with caution.[63,64]
Chemotherapy with Low-dose Radiotherapy		
Germinoma	>85% at 3 years	Life-threatening side effects include myelosuppression
Mature teratoma	—	(neutropenia and thrombocytopenia). Less severe side
Other NGGCT	—	effects are specific to the chosen chemotherapy regimen. Available data suggest a reduced incidence of adverse radiation effects, but long-term follow-up is lacking in these patients.
Surgery		
Germinoma	—	All patients should undergo stereotactic biopsy or surgical
Mature teratoma	GTR curative	tumor sampling of suspected intracranial GCTs. One
Other NGGCT	—	exception may be patients with radiographic and CSF/serum markers clearly suggestive of pure germinoma. Modern endoscopic and microsurgical techniques have reduced the risk of surgery in the pineal and suprasellar regions and there is some evidence to suggest that cytoreductive surgery may improve outcomes; however, formalized studies are needed.

High-dose radiotherapy is defined as 45 to 55 Gy to the primary tumor and 30 to 36 Gy to the craniospinal axis. Reduced-dose radiotherapy is defined as 21 to 24 Gy to the whole ventricle with a boost of 40 to 45 Gy to the primary tumor and craniospinal irradiation reserved for patients with disseminated disease. Low-dose radiotherapy indicates any regimen using lower doses of whole-ventricle and/or primary tumor radiation than those used in reduced-dose radiotherapy. Chemotherapy indicates chemotherapy-only regimens. Surgery refers to stereotactic biopsy, surgical tumor sampling, or maximal debulking as indicated. NGGCT includes embryonal carcinoma, malignant teratoma, endodermal sinus tumor, choriocarcinoma, and mixed tumors.

Abbreviations: CSF, cerebrospinal fluid; GCT, germ cell tumor; GTR, gross total resection; NGGCT, nongerminomatous germ cell tumor; PFS, progression-free survival; VP, ventriculoperitoneal; —, no data available.

overall survival rate of 27.3%, whereas patients with teratomas or mixed germinomas had a 10-year survival rate of 70.7%. One-year survival rates also varied widely with 0% survival for choriocarcinomas, 33% for endodermal sinus tumors, and 80% for embryonal carcinomas. This finding further highlights the heterogeneity of these tumors and suggests that additional studies evaluating treatment of specific tumor subtypes may improve results.

Chemotherapeutic regimens in NGGCT treatment protocols vary, but frequently include cisplatin or carboplatin and etoposide. Radiation doses are typically in the range of 30 to 36 Gy delivered to the entire craniospinal axis with a tumor boost of 20 to 54 Gy.[7,13,16,34] The rate of metastasis to the spinal cord or distant sites has been reported to be as high as 45%[13] and, unfortunately, the long-term effects of radiotherapy in these patients are of less concern given their poor overall prognosis. As a result, craniospinal irradiation is currently standard-of-care for all patients with intracranial NGGCTs. However, some investigators have suggested that spinal irradiation may not improve outcomes in patients with certain non-metastatic NGGCTs.[63,64] More research is needed to determine the role of craniospinal irradiation in the treatment of localized NGGCTs.

Although there are no definitive data to suggest that upfront gross total resection of NGGCTs improves outcomes, the frequency of mixed tumors in this group can lead to an especially high rate of diagnostic error with stereotactic biopsy.[33] This risk, coupled with the importance of accurate subtype identification for treatment and prognosis has led some investigators to suggest that the diagnostic accuracy afforded by maximal resection at the time of diagnosis is worth the inherent risks of surgery.[32] Once a diagnosis has been established, resection has been shown to play an important role in the treatment of some NGGCT subtypes. Surgical resection is the treatment of choice for mature teratomas,[32] and also plays an important role in the treatment of mixed tumors when a component of mature teratoma remains after chemotherapy and radiotherapy have been completed.[4]

In addition, surgery is the only potentially curative treatment for a distinct phenomenon first described by Logothetis and colleagues[65] in 1982 known as growing teratoma syndrome. This syndrome is characterized by rapid, paradoxic growth of a GCT—often in the setting of normalizing tumor markers—in spite of treatment with chemotherapy and radiotherapy.[66] Growing teratoma syndrome is more common in tumors outside the CNS, but has also been reported in intracranial lesions.[67–70] A recent study estimated that this phenomenon was observed in up to 21% of intracranial NGGCTs.[66] A growing teratoma is potentially curable with surgical resection and second-look surgery should be considered for any NGGCT that continues to grow in spite of adequate treatment with chemotherapy and radiotherapy.[33,66]

Surgery plays an important palliative role in the care of patients with intracranial NGGCTs who develop hydrocephalus as a result of tumor expansion. Third ventriculostomy, which involves endoscopically perforating the floor of the third ventricle to allow CSF to flow directly into the basal cisterns, is the treatment of choice for hydrocephalus in these patients unless tumor occupies the floor of the third ventricle.[32,33] Ventriculoperitoneal shunting may also be used, but has been associated with a higher complication rate[32] and an increased risk of extraneural metastasis.[54,59,60] Third ventriculostomy can easily be accomplished at the time of endoscopic tumor sampling for patients who present with obstructive hydrocephalus.[33]

The prognosis for patients with recurrent NGGCTs is extremely poor. Only 1 in 4 patients achieves full remission when relapsing after a complete response to initial therapy and very few patients who have a partial response to initial treatment achieve remission from recurrent disease.[71] Myeloablative chemotherapy with autologous hematopoietic stem cell rescue has been proposed as a potential salvage therapy for these patients. Early reports indicate that 5-year overall survival in the range of 50% may be possible using this approach.[72] The optimal chemotherapeutic regimen as well as the role of radiotherapy and surgery for recurrent NGGCTs, however, remains unclear. Future studies will also need to assess the effectiveness of myeloablative chemotherapy for specific subtypes of recurrent NGGCTs.

SUMMARY

Treatment approaches and outcomes are summarized in **Table 1**. Pure germinomas are extraordinarily radiosensitive, with complete remission rates in excess of 90% with radiation alone. The focus of treatment for these tumors, therefore, has shifted to minimizing radiation exposure to healthy tissue in an effort to reduce the risk of late sequelae including endocrine, vascular, and neurocognitive deficits. Current evidence supports reduction of whole-ventricle radiation to 21 to 24 Gy and a boost to the tumor of 40 to 45 Gy. Craniospinal irradiation can likely be reserved for patients with evidence of metastatic disease based on MRI and/or CSF cytology. Further reductions in radiation dose may be possible with the addition of neo-adjuvant chemotherapy; however, evidence is insufficient for this approach to be considered standard-of-care at this time. Recurrent disease is infrequent and salvage radiotherapy with or without chemotherapy is successful in re-inducing remission in the vast majority of patients.

NGGCTs are more refractory to radiotherapy than germinomas, and chemotherapy-only trials have proven disappointing. A combined approach offers the highest rates of remission for these patients with 5-year survival rates reported in the range of 50% to 70%. Accurate subtype diagnosis is critical, as these tumors often have mixed components. Furthermore, tumor subtype has been shown to have important implications for prognosis and treatment. Surgery plays a more prominent role in the treatment of NGGCTs than in the treatment of germinomas. Complete surgical resection of mature teratomas is curative. Third ventriculostomy plays an important role in relieving hydrocephalus secondary to tumor expansion. Second-look surgery should also be considered in patients with residual tumor after treatment with chemotherapy and radiotherapy to evaluate for a mixed teratoma component or growing tera-toma syndrome.

Intracranial GCTs are a rare and remarkably heterogeneous group of neoplasms. Although considerable advancements have been made in the diagnosis and treatment of these tumors, much remains to be learned. Specifically, the role of environmental and genetic factors in the patho-genesis may improve our understanding of tumor biology and even facilitate preventive strategies. Considerable work also remains to be done in developing and refining diagnostic and treatment approaches to intracranial GCTs. Given the young age of this patient population and the importance of radiation in the treatment of these tumors, achieving optimal outcomes will ultimately demand a careful balance of maximizing survival while mini-mizing long-term impacts on quality of life.

REFERENCES

1. Kretschmar C, Kleinberg L, Greenberg M, et al. Pre-radiation chemotherapy with response-based radiation therapy in children with central nervous system germ cell tumors: a report from the Children's Oncology Group. Pediatr Blood Cancer 2007;48: 285–91.

2. Jennings MT, Gelman R, Hochberg F. Intracranial germ-cell tumors: natural history and pathogenesis. J Neurosurg 1985;63:155–67.

3. Srinivasan N, Pakala A, Mukkamalla C, et al. Pineal germinoma. South Med J 2010;103:1031–7.

4. Friedman JA, Lynch JJ, Buckner JC, et al. Manage-ment of malignant pineal germ cell tumors with residual mature teratoma. Neurosurgery 2001;48: 518–22 [discussion: 522–3].

5. Cuccia V, Galarza M. Pure pineal germinomas: anal-ysis of gender incidence. Acta Neurochir (Wien) 2006;148:865–71 [discussion: 871].

6. Balmaceda C, Heller G, Rosenblum M, et al. Chemotherapy without irradiation—a novel approach for newly diagnosed CNS germ cell tumors: results of an international cooperative trial. The first international central nervous system germ cell tumor study. J Clin Oncol 1996;14:2908–15.

7. Calaminus G, Bamberg M, Harms D, et al. AFP/beta-HCG secreting CNS germ cell tumors: long-term outcome with respect to initial symptoms and primary tumor resection. Results of the cooperative trial MAKEI 89. Neuropediatrics 2005;36:71–7.

8. Shinoda J, Sakai N, Yano H, et al. Prognostic factors and therapeutic problems of primary intracranial choriocarcinoma/germ-cell tumors with high levels of HCG. J Neurooncol 2004;66:225–40.

9. Ogino H, Shibamoto Y, Takanaka T, et al. CNS germi-noma with elevated serum human chorionic gonado-tropin level: clinical characteristics and treatment outcome. Int J Radiat Oncol Biol Phys 2005;62:803–8.

10. Oosterhuis JW, Stoop H, Honecker F, et al. Why human extragonadal germ cell tumours occur in the midline of the body: old concepts, new perspectives. Int J Androl 2007;30:256–63 [discussion: 263–4].

11. Sano K. Pathogenesis of intracranial germ cell tumors reconsidered. J Neurosurg 1999;90:258–64.

12. Khatua S, Dhall G, O'Neil S, et al. Treatment of primary CNS germinomatous germ cell tumors with chemotherapy prior to reduced dose whole ventric-ular and local boost irradiation. Pediatr Blood Cancer 2010;55:42–6.

13. Matsutani M, Sano K, Takakura K, et al. Primary intracranial germ cell tumors: a clinical analysis of 153 histologically verified cases. J Neurosurg 1997;86:446–55.

14. Huang PI, Chen YW, Wong TT, et al. Extended focal radiotherapy of 30 Gy alone for intracranial synchro-nous bifocal germinoma: a single institute experi-ence. Childs Nerv Syst 2008;24:1315–21.

15. Lee L, Saran F, Hargrave D, et al. Germinoma with synchronous lesions in the pineal and suprasellar regions. Childs Nerv Syst 2006;22:1513–8.

16. Kyritsis AP. Management of primary intracranial germ cell tumors. J Neurooncol 2010;96:143–9.

17. Sato K, Takeuchi H, Kubota T. Pathology of intracranial germ cell tumors. Prog Neurol Surg 2009;23:59–75.

18. Haas-Kogan DA, Missett BT, Wara WM, et al. Radia-tion therapy for intracranial germ cell tumors. Int J Radiat Oncol Biol Phys 2003;56:511–8.

19. Hoffman HJ, Otsubo H, Hendrick EB, et al. Intracranial germ-cell tumors in children. J Neurosurg 1991; 74:545–51.

20. Villano JL, Virk IY, Ramirez V, et al. Descriptive epidemiology of central nervous system germ cell tumors: nonpineal analysis. Neuro Oncol 2010;12: 257–64.

21. Matsumura N, Kurimoto M, Endo S, et al. Intracranial germinoma associated with Down's syndrome. Report of 2 cases. Pediatr Neurosurg 1998;29:199–202.

22. Okada Y, Nishikawa R, Matsutani M, et al. Hypomethylated X chromosome gain and rare isochromosome 12p in diverse intracranial germ cell tumors. J Neuropathol Exp Neurol 2002;61:531–8.

23. Juric D, Sale S, Hromas RA, et al. Gene expression profiling differentiates germ cell tumors from other cancers and defines subtype-specific signatures. Proc Natl Acad Sci U S A 2005;102:17763–8.

24. Lee D, Suh YL. Histologically confirmed intracranial germ cell tumors; an analysis of 62 patients in a single institute. Virchows Arch 2010;457:347–57.

25. Packer RJ, Cohen BH, Cooney K. Intracranial germ cell tumors. Oncologist 2000;5:312–20.

26. Reisch N, Kuhne-Eversmann L, Franke D, et al. Intracranial germinoma as a very rare cause of panhypopituitarism in a 23-year old man. Exp Clin Endocrinol Diabetes 2009;117:320–3.

27. Konovalov AN, Pitskhelauri DI. Principles of treatment of the pineal region tumors. Surg Neurol 2003;59:250–68.

28. Liang L, Korogi Y, Sugahara T, et al. MRI of intracranial germ-cell tumours. Neuroradiology 2002;44:382–8.

29. Sawamura Y, de Tribolet N, Ishii N, et al. Management of primary intracranial germinomas: diagnostic surgery or radical resection? J Neurosurg 1997;87: 262–6.

30. Reddy AT, Wellons JC 3rd, Allen JC, et al. Refining the staging evaluation of pineal region germinoma using neuroendoscopy and the presence of preoperative diabetes insipidus. Neuro Oncol 2004;6: 127–33.

31. Akai T, Iizuka H, Kadoya S, et al. Extraneural metastasis of intracranial germinoma with syncytiotrophoblastic giant cells—case report. Neurol Med Chir (Tokyo) 1998;38:574–7.

32. Bruce JN, Ogden AT. Surgical strategies for treating patients with pineal region tumors. J Neurooncol 2004;69:221–36.

33. Souweidane MM, Krieger MD, Weiner HL, et al. Surgical management of primary central nervous system germ cell tumors: proceedings from the Second International Symposium on Central Nervous System Germ Cell Tumors. J Neurosurg Pediatr 2010;6:125–30.

34. Echevarria ME, Fangusaro J, Goldman S. Pediatric central nervous system germ cell tumors: a review. Oncologist 2008;13:690–9.

35. Maity A, Shu HK, Janss A, et al. Craniospinal radiation in the treatment of biopsy-proven intracranial germinomas: twenty-five years' experience in a single center. Int J Radiat Oncol Biol Phys 2004; 58:1165–70.

36. Ogawa K, Shikama N, Toita T, et al. Long-term results of radiotherapy for intracranial germinoma: a multiinstitutional retrospective review of 126 patients. Int J Radiat Oncol Biol Phys 2004;58:705–13.

37. Rogers SJ, Mosleh-Shirazi MA, Saran FH. Radiotherapy of localised intracranial germinoma: time to sever historical ties? Lancet Oncol 2005;6: 509–19.

38. Shirato H, Nishio M, Sawamura Y, et al. Analysis of long-term treatment of intracranial germinoma. Int J Radiat Oncol Biol Phys 1997;37:511–5.

39. Merchant TE, Sherwood SH, Mulhern RK, et al. CNS germinoma: disease control and long-term functional outcome for 12 children treated with craniospinal irradiation. Int J Radiat Oncol Biol Phys 2000;46: 1171–6.

40. Bamberg M, Kortmann RD, Calaminus G, et al. Radiation therapy for intracranial germinoma: results of the German cooperative prospective trials MAKEI 83/86/89. J Clin Oncol 1999;17:2585–92.

41. Shibamoto Y, Sasai K, Oya N, et al. Intracranial germinoma: radiation therapy with tumor volume-based dose selection. Radiology 2001;218:452–6.

42. Yen SH, Chen YW, Huang PI, et al. Optimal treatment for intracranial germinoma: can we lower radiation dose without chemotherapy? Int J Radiat Oncol Biol Phys 2010;77:980–7.

43. Sawamura Y, Ikeda J, Shirato H, et al. Germ cell tumours of the central nervous system: treatment consideration based on 111 cases and their long-term clinical outcomes. Eur J Cancer 1998;34: 104–10.

44. Sugiyama K, Yamasaki F, Kurisu K, et al. Quality of life of extremely long-time germinoma survivors mainly treated with radiotherapy. Prog Neurol Surg 2009;23:130–9.

45. Sands SA, Kellie SJ, Davidow AL, et al. Long-term quality of life and neuropsychologic functioning for patients with CNS germ-cell tumors: from the First International CNS Germ-Cell Tumor Study. Neuro Oncol 2001;3:174–83.

46. Buckner JC, Peethambaram PP, Smithson WA, et al. Phase II trial of primary chemotherapy followed by reduced-dose radiation for CNS germ cell tumors. J Clin Oncol 1999;17:933–40.

47. Endo H, Kumabe T, Jokura H, et al. Stereotactic radiosurgery followed by whole ventricular irradiation for primary intracranial germinoma of the pineal region. Minim Invasive Neurosurg 2005;48:186–90.

48. Kawabata Y, Takahashi JA, Arakawa Y, et al. Long term outcomes in patients with intracranial germinomas: a single institution experience of irradiation

with or without chemotherapy. J Neurooncol 2008; 88:161–7.

49. Nguyen QN, Chang EL, Allen PK, et al. Focal and craniospinal irradiation for patients with intracranial germinoma and patterns of failure. Cancer 2006; 107:2228–36.

50. Cho J, Choi JU, Kim DS, et al. Low-dose craniospinal irradiation as a definitive treatment for intracranial germinoma. Radiother Oncol 2009;91:75–9.

51. Haddock MG, Schild SE, Scheithauer BW, et al. Radiation therapy for histologically confirmed primary central nervous system germinoma. Int J Radiat Oncol Biol Phys 1997;38:915–23.

52. Wenger M, Lovblad KO, Markwalder R, et al. Late recurrence of pineal germinoma. Surg Neurol 2002;57:34–9 [discussion: 39–40].

53. da Silva NS, Cappellano AM, Diez B, et al. Primary chemotherapy for intracranial germ cell tumors: results of the third international CNS germ cell tumor study. Pediatr Blood Cancer 2010;54:377–83.

54. Ono N, Isobe I, Uki J, et al. Recurrence of primary intracranial germinomas after complete response with radiotherapy: recurrence patterns and therapy. Neurosurgery 1994;35:615–20 [discussion: 620–1].

55. Regine WF, Hodes JE, Patchell RA. Intracranial germinoma: treatment with radiosurgery alone—a case report. J Neurooncol 1998;37:75–7.

56. Casentini L, Colombo F, Pozza F, et al. Combined radiosurgery and external radiotherapy of intracranial germinomas. Surg Neurol 1990;34:79–86.

57. Kellie SJ, Boyce H, Dunkel IJ, et al. Intensive cisplatin and cyclophosphamide-based chemotherapy without radiotherapy for intracranial germinomas: failure of a primary chemotherapy approach. Pediatr Blood Cancer 2004;43:126–33.

58. Bouffet E, Baranzelli MC, Patte C, et al. Combined treatment modality for intracranial germinomas: results of a multicentre SFOP experience. Societe Francaise d'Oncologie Pediatrique. Br J Cancer 1999;79:1199–204.

59. Howman-Giles R, Besser M, Johnston IH, et al. Disseminated hematogenous metastases from a pineal germinoma in an infant. Case report. J Neurosurg 1984;60:835–7.

60. Pallini R, Bozzini V, Scerrati M, et al. Bone metastasis associated with shunt-related peritoneal deposits from a pineal germinoma. Case report and review of the literature. Acta Neurochir (Wien) 1991;109:78–83.

61. Fuller BG, Kapp DS, Cox R. Radiation therapy of pineal region tumors: 25 new cases and a review of 208 previously reported cases. Int J Radiat Oncol Biol Phys 1994;28:229–45.

62. Kochi M, Itoyama Y, Shiraishi S, et al. Successful treatment of intracranial nongerminomatous malignant germ cell tumors by administering neoadjuvant chemotherapy and radiotherapy before excision of residual tumors. J Neurosurg 2003;99:106–14.

63. Smith AA, Weng E, Handler M, et al. Intracranial germ cell tumors: a single institution experience and review of the literature. J Neurooncol 2004;68: 153–9.

64. Ushio Y, Kochi M, Kuratsu J, et al. Preliminary observations for a new treatment in children with primary intracranial yolk sac tumor or embryonal carcinoma. Report of five cases. J Neurosurg 1999;90:133–7.

65. Logothetis CJ, Samuels ML, Trindade A, et al. The growing teratoma syndrome. Cancer 1982;50: 1629–35.

66. Kim CY, Choi JW, Lee JY, et al. Intracranial growing teratoma syndrome: clinical characteristics and treatment strategy. J Neurooncol 2011; 101:109–15.

67. Hanna A, Edan C, Heresbach N, et al. Expanding mature pineal teratoma syndrome. Case report. Neurochirurgie 2000;46:568–72 [in French].

68. Lee AC, Chan GC, Fung CF, et al. Paradoxical response of a pineal immature teratoma to combination chemotherapy. Med Pediatr Oncol 1995;24: 53–7.

69. O'Callaghan AM, Katapodis O, Ellison DW, et al. The growing teratoma syndrome in a nongerminomatous germ cell tumor of the pineal gland: a case report and review. Cancer 1997;80:942–7.

70. Yagi K, Kageji T, Nagahiro S, et al. Growing teratoma syndrome in a patient with a non-germinomatous germ cell tumor in the neurohypophysis—case report. Neurol Med Chir (Tokyo) 2004;44:33–7.

71. Motzer RJ, Mazumdar M, Bosl GJ, et al. High-dose carboplatin, etoposide, and cyclophosphamide for patients with refractory germ cell tumors: treatment results and prognostic factors for survival and toxicity. J Clin Oncol 1996;14:1098–105.

72. Bouffet E. The role of myeloablative chemotherapy with autologous hematopoietic cell rescue in central nervous system germ cell tumors. Pediatr Blood Cancer 2010;54:644–6.

Pediatric Considerations for Pineal Tumor Management

E.J. Fontana, MD[a],*, J. Garvin, MD[b], N. Feldstein, MD[a], R.C.E. Anderson, MD[a]

KEYWORDS

• Pineal tumor • Germ cell • Pediatric • Hydrocephalus

Pineal region tumors are rare, accounting for 0.4% of tumors found in the central nervous system (CNS).[1] Pineal region tumors are nearly 10 times more common in the pediatric population than in adults, accounting for 2.8% to 9% of all childhood CNS malignancies.[2,3] There are 3 main categories of pediatric pineal region tumors based on histology and cell origin: germ cell tumors (GCTs), pineal parenchymal tumors, and others, which include tumors of glial cell origin and rare metastases. Of these, GCTs are the most common, representing 50% to 75% of all pediatric pineal region tumors, depending on the study. Pineal parenchymal tumors are the second most common, representing 15% to 30%,[4,5] and other tumors, such as astrocytoma, ependymoma, lymphoma, and atypical teratoid rhabdoid tumors, are less common.

Demographics of the affected pediatric population vary depending on histologic diagnosis. Pineal region GCTs occur almost exclusively in boys aged 10 to 19 years and have a marked increased prevalence in the Asian population, notably in Japan and Korea. GCTs may be associated with Klinefelter syndrome. Pineal parenchymal tumors occur with equal frequency in both genders, with one study citing a mean age of 12 years.[6]

Several studies have looked at the histologic breakdown of pineal tumors within the pediatric population (**Table 1**). Among GCTs, about 60% are pure germinomas, and the remainder are nongerminomatous GCTs (NGGCTs), including yolk sac tumor (endodermal sinus tumor), choriocarcinoma, embryonal carcinoma, and mixed malignant GCTs (comprising germinoma or teratoma with additional malignant elements). Pineal parenchymal tumors include pineocytoma, a benign lesion, and pineoblastoma, a World Health Organization grade IV malignant primitive neuroectodermal tumor (PNET).

Overall treatment strategies for these tumors vary significantly depending on histologic diagnosis and continue to evolve as new techniques become available. Treatment of malignant pineal tumors generally involves surgical resection or biopsy, radiation therapy, and chemotherapy. For symptomatic benign tumors, such as pineocytomas, pineal cysts, pilocytic astrocytomas, and mature teratomas, surgical resection is the definitive therapy. Surgery generally plays a role in the management of nearly all these patients because of the need for tissue diagnosis and management of hydrocephalus. In addition, there is growing evidence to support aggressive debulking of malignant lesions to improve efficacy of adjuvant therapies.[6]

This article discusses current strategies for preoperative evaluation, operative management, and postoperative care of the pediatric patient with a newly diagnosed pineal region tumor.

[a] Department of Neurological Surgery, Neurological Institute, Columbia University Medical Center, New York, NY 10036, USA
[b] Department of Oncology, Morgan Stanley Children's Hospital of New York, Columbia University Medical Center, New York, NY 10036, USA
* Corresponding author.
E-mail address: ejf2024@columbia.edu

Neurosurg Clin N Am 22 (2011) 395–402
doi:10.1016/j.nec.2011.05.003

Table 1
The predominance of GCTs among pineal region tumors. In all 3 studies shown, GCTs comprise more than one-third, and in most cases more than two-thirds of all pineal region tumors in children

Study	N	Age Range (y)	Histologic Breakdown, n (%)
Al-Hussaini et al[35]	355	0–18	GCT, 237 (67) PPT, 96 (27) Glioma, 9 (2) AT/RT, 2 (<1) Other, 11 (3)
Yazici et al[36]	24	0.5–15.1	Germinoma, 5 (21) NGGCT, 4 (17) PPT, 10 (42) Glioma, 1 (4) Other, 4 (17)
Cho et al[9]	35	0–20	Germinoma, 10 (28.5) NGGCT, 19 (54) PPT, 8 (22.8) Glioma, 3 (8.6)

Abbreviations: AT/RT, atypical rhabdoid/teratoid tumor; NGGCT, nongerminomatous GCT; PPT, pineal parenchymal tumor.

PREOPERATIVE ASSESSMENT

There are 3 main mechanisms by which pineal tumors become symptomatic: elevated intracranial pressure from obstructive hydrocephalus, direct compression of the brainstem or cerebellum, and neuroendocrine dysfunction.[7] The most common presenting symptoms seen in patients with pineal lesions are related to hydrocephalus. Symptoms reported include headache, Parinaud syndrome, decreased visual acuity, ataxia, and diabetes insipidus. Less-frequent symptoms include precocious puberty and hypogonadism.[8] In 2 studies by Mandera and colleagues[6] and Cho,[9] the mean duration of symptoms was between 5 and 10 months, respectively. Symptoms often correlate with the degree of hydrocephalus, and in the study by Cho, 29 of 48 patients had moderate to severe hydrocephalus on imaging that warranted immediate cerebrospinal fluid (CSF) diversion.[9]

Head computed tomography (CT) or brain magnetic resonance imaging (MRI) typically demonstrate a lesion within the posterior portion of the third ventricle, protruding anteroinferiorly to the tectal plate. It is difficult to differentiate between GCTs and pineal parenchymal tumors based on imaging alone. Pineal gland calcification is commonly seen in all types of pineal tumors and cannot typically aid in diagnosis. Findings on CT are generally isodense to hyperdense lesions that are contrast enhancing. On MRI, lesions may be isointense to hypointense on T1-weighted imaging and may vary from isointense to hyperintense on T2-weighted imaging. The tumors are most often heterogeneously enhancing (**Figs. 1** and **2**). Because of possible synchronous lesions, total neuroaxis imaging is recommended. Disease dissemination may occur intracranially, most commonly in the pituitary region or thalamus, and is most frequently associated with GCTs (**Fig. 3**).[8] One study estimated that one-third of patients show spinal dissemination at the time of diagnosis,[10] with other study estimates ranging from 10% to 57%.[7]

In all patients presenting with a newly diagnosed pineal region tumor, appropriate initial workup includes MRI of the brain and total spine with and without contrast, evaluation of serum markers for α-fetoprotein, β-human chorionic gonadotropin

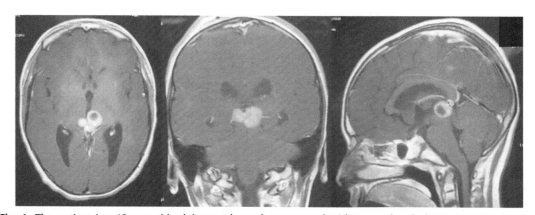

Fig. 1. The patient is a 13-year-old adolescent boy who presented with severe headaches and vomiting after several weeks of worsening headaches and Parinaud syndrome. Imaging revealed a pineal region mass with obstructive hydrocephalus. Frozen tissue biopsy diagnosis was germinoma, and the patient was treated successfully with radiation and chemotherapy.

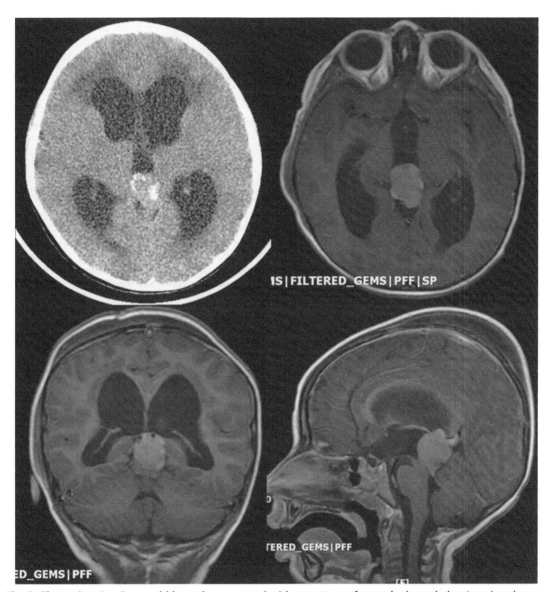

Fig. 2. The patient is a 3-year-old boy who presented with symptoms of acute hydrocephalus. Imaging demonstrated obstructive hydrocephalus from a pineal region mass. Biopsy revealed a diagnosis of pineoblastoma, and a complete surgical resection was performed followed by adjuvant radiation and chemotherapy.

(β-hCG), routine laboratory tests to rule out metabolic abnormalities or infection, evaluation for endocrine dysfunction, and CSF diversion with either placement of an external ventricular drain or an endoscopic third ventriculostomy (ETV) if hydrocephalus is present. CSF should additionally be tested for germ cell markers as well as cytology. Preoperative CSF sampling is a critical part of the workup because CSF has greater sensitivity than serum and may be diagnostic. Elevation of CSF α-fetoprotein levels above 10 ng/mL and/or β-hCG above 50 mIU/mL is diagnostic of NGGCT; isolated lesser elevation of β-hCG levels may occur in pure germinoma. In addition to diagnostic

purposes, lumbar CSF is also important in determining postoperative chemotherapy protocol eligibility. Except for patients in whom elevated serum or CSF marker levels are diagnostic for endodermal sinus tumor or choriocarcinoma, histopathologic diagnosis must be made by tissue biopsy.

SURGICAL TREATMENT

In patients with obstructive hydrocephalus, CSF diversion is frequently planned before resection of tumor. Options for CSF diversion include placement of external ventricular drain, ventriculoperitoneal shunt, and ETV. However, ETV is generally the

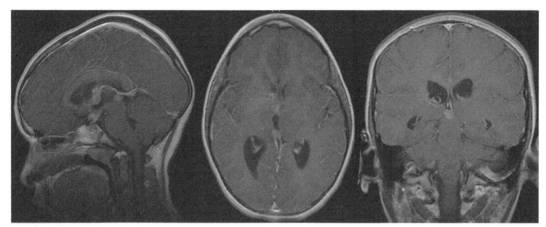

Fig. 3. The patient is a 16-year-old adolescent girl who presented to the emergency room with diabetes insipidus and 1 month of ataxia, headaches, and vomiting. Imaging revealed synchronous lesions in the pineal region, hypothalamus, and septum causing obstruction of the foramen of Monro. CSF studies revealed elevated β-hCG and normal α-fetoprotein levels. A presumptive diagnosis of germinoma was made based on CSF markers and imaging, and the patient went on to receive chemotherapy and radiation with good response.

preferred choice in patients requiring treatment for hydrocephalus before tumor resection.[11–13] Reasons for this include higher risks of infection, increased tumor dissemination, shunt failure, overshunting, and subdural hematoma associated with ventriculoperitoneal shunt placement.

When the decision is made to perform an initial biopsy, the biopsy may be performed via an endoscopic, stereotactic, or open approach. Biopsy enables tissue diagnosis for the planning of adjuvant therapy without open resection. In addition, biopsy guides the surgeon in the decision to perform radical tumor resection. Several recent studies have advocated the use of endoscopy for biopsy over the stereotactic approach and report a histologic diagnosis in 75% to 94% of tumors biopsied.[14–16] These results are comparable with biopsy yields previously reported for stereotactic biopsy of between 87% and 97%,[17,18] and endoscopic approach offers the additional benefit of simultaneous ETV as well as visualization of the lesion at the time of biopsy. Wong and colleagues[11] advocate the use of endoscopy to simultaneously perform ETV and tumor biopsy in patients with obstructive hydrocephalus before performing radical resection. In their study, histologic diagnosis was achieved in 21 of 25 (84%) patients who underwent endoscopic tumor biopsy. Endoscopy also does not need to be limited to patients with ventriculomegaly. A recent study by Naftel and colleagues[19] describes successful biopsy of tumors in patients with small ventricles with low morbidity and high diagnostic yield. In this report, a brain navigation system was used for initial trajectory into the ventricle. A 1.1-mm endoscope (NeuroPEN, Medtronic) was used inside a 1.7-mm

ventricular catheter, and 10 to 20 mL of lactated Ringer solution was insufflated into the ventricle to improve visualization. Postoperatively, an external ventricular drain was left in case of need for emergent CSF diversion, although no patient from this group ultimately required additional CSF diversion procedures. Bruce and colleagues[7] have described the role of stereotactic biopsy in determining the need for total resection. This approach is particularly appropriate if CSF diversion has already been established or in patients without hydrocephalus. Stereotactic biopsy does not confer the same opportunity to perform simultaneous ETV, but it is equally safe and likely to yield diagnostic tissue.

A third option for obtaining tissue is open resection. Because aggressive surgical resection of benign pineal region tumors as well as many malignant lesions affords the best outcome for the patient, open biopsy is the approach favored at the authors' institution for patients with negative CSF and serum markers.[16,20–22] In addition, because there is often significant heterogeneity seen in germ cell histology, open biopsy is more likely to yield accurate histologic diagnosis (**Fig. 4**).[7] General indications for surgery include symptomatic benign lesions for which surgery is curative, cytoreduction of tumor for chemotherapy/radiotherapy of malignant lesions, and removal of residual tumor after chemotherapy.[11] Whenever possible, if the patient is going to undergo biopsy, we perform an open biopsy with a plan to resect the lesion after frozen tissue is obtained. Once frozen specimen is obtained, surgical resection can be performed, unless the frozen specimen yields a diagnosis of germinoma, in

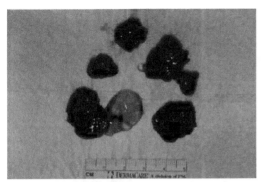

Fig. 4. Gross pathology showing mixed GCT with significant heterogeneity. Such heterogeneity can lead to misdiagnosis if tissue sampling is limited.

which case no further surgery is indicated. For patients undergoing planned surgical resection of a pineal region tumor, operative approaches include the supracerebellar-infratentorial (SCIT) approach, the occipital-transtentorial (OTT) approach, and the transcallosal-interhemispheric approach.[11] In the pediatric population, the SCIT and OTT approaches may be performed in modified prone, park bench, or sitting position.[23] The authors favor the sitting position and have successfully used this position in children as young as 2 years (**Fig. 5**). When planning a surgical resection, it is important to consider the anatomic relationship of the tumor with the third ventricle, tentorium, falx, and vein of Galen. Preoperative MRI can usually provide this information.

Although less frequently used, the OTT approach provides good access to the superior third ventricle and tentorial apex. Using an OTT approach, the patient is typically placed in a sitting position with the head in a moderate degree of flexion. Typically, a horseshoe incision is made on the right nondominant side, and the craniotomy is performed to expose the posterior portion of the superior sagittal sinus at the upper edge of the torcula. Once the brain is exposed, the occipital lobe is retracted superolaterally to visualize the tentorium. The tentorium is then dissected parallel to the straight sinus to allow access to the tumor.[24] The SCIT approach provides the best access for midline tumors, which are primarily inferior to the tentorium, and may limit access to tumors that extend far laterally. The patient is again typically placed in a sitting position, which provides the advantage of gravity dropping the cerebellum and providing 1 to 2 cm of space between the superior surface of the cerebellum and the tentorium. This approach can be used even in patients with a steeply angled tentorium, provided the neck is supple enough to enable adequate flexion during positioning (**Fig. 6**). There is generally less traction required using the SCIT approach, particularly when performed in the sitting position. This approach uses a midline incision and bilateral craniotomy extending from the inferior margins of the transverse sinuses to the rim of the foramen magnum. Both approaches avoid splitting of the vermis, an important consideration in the pediatric population because of its association with postoperative mutism. In the case of extremely large tumors, the surgeon can also use both OTT and SCIT approaches to attain complete resection.

Perioperative management should include intravenous steroids with antacid or proton pump inhibitors to prevent ulcer formation. Antibiotics should be given before skin incision and are typically continued for 24 hours postoperatively or for coverage if an external ventricular drain is left

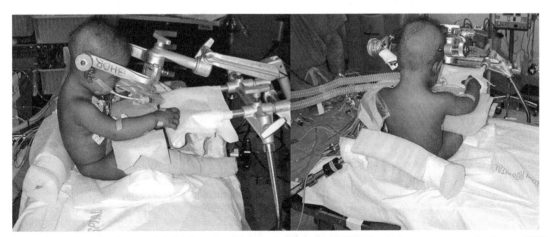

Fig. 5. The patient is a 3-year-old girl found to have a pineal region PNET. The lesion was removed using an SCIT surgical approach in the sitting position. A Layla bar (NMT Neurosciences, Ruggles Instrumentation, Madison, WI, USA) was used to support the arms, and a Mayfield (Ohio Medical Instrument Co, Cincinatti, OH, USA) with pediatric pins was used for positioning the head.

A   **B**

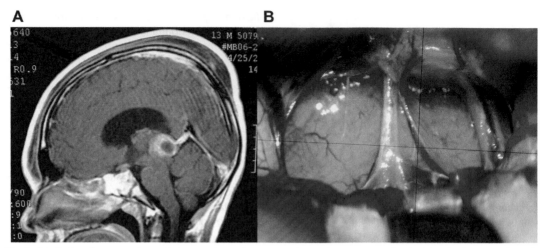

Fig. 6. (A, B) Despite a steeply angled tentorium, the tumor pictured was approached with a SCIT approach in the sitting position. This enabled good visualization with minimal retraction.

postoperatively. In these cases, antibiotics are often continued until removal of the drain. Patients should be monitored in the intensive care unit, with the primary concern being the risk of developing acute hydrocephalus. Prophylactic anticonvulsants are generally not required.

POSTOPERATIVE TREATMENT

Pineal tumors remain a relatively rare entity, a factor that has led to somewhat variable treatment strategies. However, most studies advocate the use of surgery as well as adjuvant chemotherapy and radiation therapy. Treatment strategies for pineal region tumors are best divided into 2 broad categories: treatment of GCTs and treatment of pineal parenchymal tumors.

Irradiation remains the initial treatment of choice for pure germinomas and is often curative in these patients.[14,25] Patients with disseminated disease are treated with craniospinal irradiation (CSI, 30–36 Gy) and an additional 15-Gy boost to the primary site. Recent studies suggest that CSI may not be necessary in patients with localized disease, which may help to reduce the side effects of cognitive decline and endocrine dysfunction often seen after CSI in these children.[2] Smaller volumes, such as whole brain or whole ventricle with doses of 45 to 50 Gy, result in 10-year survival exceeding 80%. Chemotherapy-alone regimens have had unacceptably high failure rates in children,[26] leading to trials of combined lower-dose radiotherapy and chemotherapy to maximize outcome survival while reducing radiation side effects. Dhall and colleagues[2] report a protocol of 4 cycles of chemotherapy with carboplatin and etoposide followed by 30-Gy total dose of

radiation with a 3-year progression-free survival (PFS) of 89.5%. As with germinomas, radiation plays an important role in the treatment of NGGCT. The Children's Oncology Group trial, ACNS0122, treated patients with 36-Gy CSI after 6 cycles of carboplatin/etoposide alternating with ifosfamide/etoposide and achieved a projected survival of 93.3%.[27] Similar outcomes were seen in the results of a Japanese GCT study group trial with a similar protocol of 5 cycles of carboplatin/etoposide followed by 54-Gy irradiation to the tumor bed.[28]

In the treatment of pineoblastoma, reported outcomes vary according to patient age. For children older than 3 years treated with radiation and chemotherapy, 5-year PFS ranges from 54% to 76%.[2] For children younger than 3 years, treatment strategies have favored chemotherapy alone because of the deleterious effects of radiation to the developing brain. However, with chemotherapy alone or chemotherapy and deferred irradiation, the 5-year PFS is considerably worse than in older children, ranging from 0% to 9%. An alternative approach of intensive chemotherapy followed by consolidative myeloablative chemotherapy with autologous hematopoietic progenitor cell rescue yielded 15% PFS.[29–37]

SUMMARY

Pineal tumors are relatively rare CNS lesions with a predilection for the pediatric population. Establishing an accurate histologic diagnosis is critical for effective treatment of these tumors. Although NGGCTs may be diagnosed via CSF markers without biopsy, most lesions require surgery for a biopsy to obtain tissue diagnosis. The biopsy can be done open, using stereotaxis, or with endoscopy. Patients also frequently suffer from hydrocephalus that can be treated emergently or at the time of biopsy or tumor resection. For GCTs, biopsy is sufficient, given the predicted good response to radiotherapy and chemotherapy. Aggressive tumor resection is indicated for pineal PNET and other non-GCT malignant lesions, and surgery should typically be followed by CSI and chemotherapy (PNET) or involved field irradiation (ependymoma, astrocytoma). For very young children with pineal PNET, the outcome with radiation and chemotherapy has been poor, and newer approaches are being applied, including intensive chemotherapy with consolidative myeloablative chemotherapy and autologous hematopoietic progenitor cell rescue.

REFERENCES

1. CBTRUS (2007–2008). Statistical report: primary brain tumors in the United States. Central Brain Tumor Registry of the United States. Available at: http://www.cbtrus.org. Accessed May 5, 2011.

2. Dhall G, Khatua S, Finlay J. Pineal region tumors in children. Curr Opin Neurol 2010;23(6):576–82.

3. The Committee of Brain Tumor Registry of Japan. Report of brain tumor registry of Japan (1969–1996). Part 1: general features of brain tumors. Neurol Med Chir (Tokyo) 2003;43(Suppl:i–vii):1–25.

4. Hirato J, Nakazato Y. Pathology of pineal region tumors. J Neurooncol 2001;54:239–49.

5. Louis DN, Ohgaki H, Wiestler OD, et al. Tumors of the pineal region. WHO classification of tumors of the central nervous system. Lyon (France): IARC Press; 2007. p. 121–6.

6. Mandera M, Marcol W, Kotulska K. Childhood pineal parenchymal tumors: clinical and therapeutic aspects. Neurosurg Rev 2010;34(2):191–6.

7. Anderson RC, Bruce J. Current management of germinomas. Contemporary Neurosurgery 2003;25(6):1–7.

8. Nagaishi M, Suzuki R, Tanaka Y, et al. Pure germinomas of the pineal gland with synchronous spinal dissemination. Neurol Med Chir 2010;50:505–8.

9. Cho BK, Wang KC, Nam DH. Pineal tumors: experience with 48 cases over 10 years. Childs Nerv Syst 1998;14(102):53–8.

10. Drevelegas A, Strigaris AK, Samara CH. Pineal tumors, imaging of brain tumors with histological correlations. 2nd edition. Berlin: Springer; 2011. p. 201–13.

11. Wong TT, Chen HH, Liang ML, et al. Neuroendoscopy in the management of pineal tumors. Childs Nerv Syst 2011;27(6):949–59.

12. Bruce JN, Ogden AT. Surgical strategies for treating patients with pineal region tumors. J Neurooncol 2004;69(1–3):221–36.

13. Goodman R. Magnetic resonance imaging-directed stereotactic endoscopic third ventriculostomy. Neurosurgery 1993;32:1043–7.

14. Maity A, Shu HK, Janss A, et al. Craniospinal radiation in the treatment of biopsy proven intracranial germinomas: twenty-five years' experience in a single center. Int J Radiat Oncol Biol Phys 2004; 58:1165–70.

15. Kumar SV, Mohanty A, Santosh V, et al. Endoscopic options in management of posterior third ventricular tumors. Childs Nerv Syst 2007;23:1135–45.

16. Al-Tamimi YZ, Bhargava D, Surash S, et al. Endoscopic biopsy during third ventriculostomy of pediatric pineal region tumors. Childs Nerv Syst 2008; 24:1323–6.

17. Pople IK, Athanasiou TC, Sandeman DR, et al. The role of endoscopic biopsy and third ventriculostomy in the management of pineal region tumours. Br J Neurosurg 2001;15(4):305–11.

18. Kreth FW, Schatz CR, Pagenstecher A, et al. Stereotactic management of lesions of the pineal region. Neurosurgery 1996;39(2):280–9 [discussion: 9–91].

19. Naftel RP, Shannon CN, Reed GT, et al. Small-ventricle neuroendoscopy for pediatric brain tumor management. J Neurosurg Pediatr 2011;7:104–10.

20. Bruce JN. Pineal tumors. In: Winn H, editor. Youman's neurological surgery. Philadelphia: WB Saunders; 2004. p. 1011–29.

21. Stein BM, Bruce JN. Surgical management of pineal region tumors honored guest lecture. Clin Neurosurg 1992;39:509–32.

22. Weiner HL, Finlay JL. Surgery in the management of primary intracranial germ cell tumors. Childs Nerv Syst 1999;15(11–12):770–3.

23. Chen L, Mao Y. Consensus and controversies on pineal tumor surgery. World Neurosurg 2010;74(4–5): 446–7.

24. Souweidane MM. Endoscopic surgery for intraventricular brain tumors in patients without hydrocephalus. Neurosurgery 2008;62(6 Suppl 3): SHC1042–8.

25. Lutterbach J, Fauchon F, Schild SE, et al. Malignant pineal parenchymal tumors in adult patients: patterns of care and prognostic factors. Neurosurgery 2002;51(1):44–55 [discussion: 6].

26. da Silva NS, Cappellano AM, Diez B, et al. Primary chemotherapy for intracranial germ cell tumors: results of the third international CNS germ cell tumor study. Pediatr Blood Cancer 2010;54:377–83.

27. Huang P-I, Chen YW, Wong TT, et al. Extended focal radiotherapy of 30 Gy alone for intracranial synchronous bifocal germinoma: single institute experience. Childs Nerv Syst 2008;24:315–21.

28. Goldman S, Bouffet E, Fisher G, et al. A phase II trial of neoadjuvant chemotherapy +/– second-look surgery prior to radiotherapy for nongerminomatous germ cell tumors: Children's Oncology Group Study

ACNS0122 [abstract: GCT 06]. Neuro-oncology 2010;12:ii29.

29. Fangusaro J, Finlay J, Sposto R, et al. Intensive chemotherapy followed by consolidative myeloablative chemotherapy with autologous hematopoietic cell rescue (AuHCR) in young children with newly diagnosed supratentorial primitive neuroectodermal tumors (sPNET): report of the Head Start I and II experience. Pediatr Blood Cancer 2008;50:312–8.

30. Schild SE, Scheithauer BW, Haddock MG, et al. Histologically confirmed pineal tumors and other germ cell tumors of the brain. Cancer 1996;78(12): 2564–71.

31. Cuccia V. Pinealoblastomas in children. Childs Nerv Syst 2006;22(6):577–85.

32. Regis J, Bouillot P, Rouby-Volot F, et al. Pineal region tumors and the role of stereotactic biopsy: review of the mortality, morbidity, and diagnostic rates in 370 cases. Neurosurgery 1996;39(5):907–12 [discussion: 12–4].

33. Matsutani M. Excellent 10-year's OS & PFS of patients with non germinomatous germ cell tumors treated by surgery, radiation and chemotherapy. Neuro-oncology 2010;12:ii28 [abstract: GCT 03].

34. Al-Hussaini M, Sultan I, Abuirmileh N, et al. Pineal gland tumors: experience from the SEER database. J Neurooncol 2009;94:351–8.

35. Yazici N, Varan A, Soylemezoglu F, et al. Pineal region tumors in children: a single center experience. Neuropediatrics 2009;40(1):15–21.

36. Korogi Y. MRI of pineal region tumors. J Neurooncol 2001;54:251–61.

37. Geyer JR, Sposto R, Jennings M, et al. Multiagent chemotherapy and deferred radiotherapy in infants with malignant brain tumors: a report from the Children's Cancer Group. J Clin Oncol 2005;23:7621–31.

Contemporary Management of Pineocytoma

Aaron J. Clark, MD, PhD[a], Michael E. Sughrue, MD[b], Derick Aranda, MD[a], Andrew T. Parsa, MD, PhD[a],*

KEYWORDS

- Pineocytoma • Surgery • Radiotherapy
- Gross total resection • Tumor control • Overall survival

Pineocytoma is a rare tumor, accounting for 0.4% to 1% of all intracranial tumors.[1] The literature is primarily composed to case reports and small case series, occasionally with pineocytoma analyzed together with pineal region tumors of varying histology and behavior. Consequently, reported outcomes have traditionally varied, with tumor control rates ranging from 67% to 100%.[2,3] These outcomes are based on a variety of treatment modalities, including aggressive resection, subtotal resection, radiotherapy, radiosurgery, or chemotherapy.[4–7] Therefore, generating definitive treatment goals and guidelines has been difficult. The authors recently systematically reviewed the existing literature on pineocytoma to generate treatment recommendations based on specific outcomes.[8,9] This review comprised 64 publications describing 168 patients.[4–68]

SURGICAL DEBULKING IMPROVES TUMOR CONTROL AND SURVIVAL

The pineal region harbors tumors of diverse pathology, and therefore obtaining a definitive tissue diagnosis is the initial goal of surgery.[69] Open biopsy in generally preferred relative to stereotactic biopsy for tumors in this location.[70] Because of the unique location of the pineal gland with respect to the vein of Galen as it receives the basal vein of Rosenthal, the internal cerebral, and the inferior occipital veins, the benefits of any open surgical procedure in this area must be weighted against risk to these critical deep venous structures.[71,72] These structures will be encountered regardless of approach selection. The authors showed that, in the setting of pineocytoma, surgical resection reduced the overall reported rate of progression compared with biopsy (6.3% vs 17.8%; χ^2 $P<.05$).[8] The 1- and 5-year progression-free survival rates for the surgical resection group versus the biopsy group were 97% versus 90%, and 89% versus 75%, respectively, which represented a statistically significant improvement on Kaplan-Meier analysis (log-rank, $P<.05$) (**Fig. 1**A). When comparing surgical resection versus biopsy, the 1- and 5-year overall survival rates were 89% versus 82%, and 76% versus 64%, respectively.[9] Although the trend was toward improved survival with surgical resection, this difference did not reach statistical significance (log-rank, $P = .19$) (see **Fig. 1**B). Thus, despite a suggestion of benefit, the data are insufficient to definitively conclude that surgical resection provides a survival benefit over a biopsy procedure combined with adjuvant therapy. Nevertheless, once committed to an open craniotomy to obtain a tissue diagnosis, tumor debulking should be attempted if the diagnosis is pineocytoma.[73]

The authors have nothing to disclose.
[a] Department of Neurological Surgery, University of California, San Francisco, 505 Parnassus Avenue, M779, Box 0112, San Francisco, CA 94117, USA
[b] Comprehensive Brain Tumor Center, Department of Neurological Surgery, University of Oklahoma, 1000 North Lincoln Boulevard, Suite 400, Oklahoma City, OK 73104-5023, USA
* Corresponding author.
E-mail address: parsaa@neurosurg.ucsf.edu

Neurosurg Clin N Am 22 (2011) 403–407
doi:10.1016/j.nec.2011.05.004
1042-3680/11/$ – see front matter © 2011 Published by Elsevier Inc.

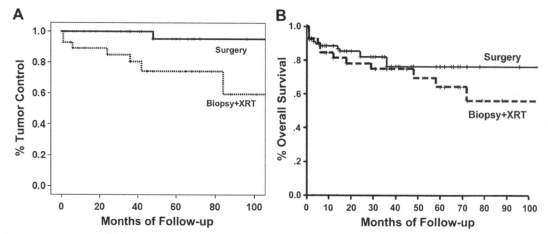

Fig. 1. Comparison of (*A*) progression-free survival and (*B*) overall survival among patients treated with surgical resection (*solid line*) versus biopsy (*dashed line*).

GROSS TOTAL RESECTION IMPROVES TUMOR CONTROL AND SURVIVAL

Aggressive surgery attempted in the pineal region carries the risk of devastating postoperative neurologic deterioration.[74] Risk/benefit analyses based on outcomes data must be considered preoperatively. For the diagnosis of pineocytoma, no tumor recurrence was reported in patients who underwent gross total resection, which represented a significant improvement over patients receiving subtotal resection plus radiation (0% vs 9.5%, respectively; χ^2 $P<.05$).[8] The 1- and 5-year progression-free survival rates for the surgical resection group versus the biopsy group was 100% versus 94%, and 100% versus 84%, respectively, which represented a statistically significant improvement on Kaplan-Meier analysis (log-rank, $P<.05$) (**Fig. 2**A). The 1- and 5-year overall survival rates for the gross total resection group

versus the subtotal resection plus radiation (subtotal resection plus radiotherapy) group was 91% versus 88%, and 84% versus 17%, respectively.[9] On Kaplan-Meier analysis, these differences represented a statistically significant improvement (log-rank, $P<.05$) (see **Fig.** 2B). When compared with gross total resection, the addition of adjuvant radiotherapy to subtotal resection does not seem to provide an equivalent tumor control or survival outcome. Therefore, despite the difficult location of pineocytoma and the associated inherent surgical risks, aggressive resection should be undertaken, because gross total resection can be potentially curative.

ADJUVANT RADIOTHERAPY DOES NOT IMPROVE TUMOR CONTROL OR SURVIVAL

Limited data suggest a role for fractionated radiotherapy in pineocytoma management.[75] Although

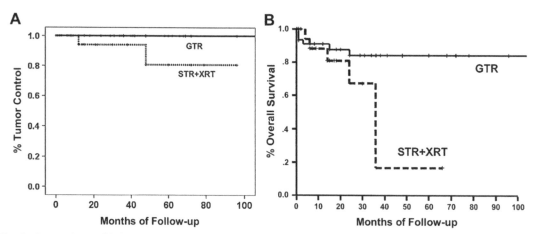

Fig. 2. Comparison of (*A*) progression-free survival and (*B*) overall survival among patients treated with gross total resection (*solid line*) versus subtotal resection plus radiotherapy (*dashed line*).

the authors' data show that gross total resection should be aggressively pursued to improve tumor control rates and extend survival, complete removal may not always be possible. In this setting, what is the role of adjuvant radiotherapy? In patients with pineocytoma, subtotal resection alone was associated with a similar rate of recurrence compared with treatment with subtotal resection plus radiotherapy (7.7% vs 11%; χ^2 P = .86). The 1- and 5-year progression-free survival rates for the subtotal resection groups versus the subtotal resection plus radiotherapy group were 100% and 94% (1-year), and 100% and 81% (5-year), respectively, which were not significantly different according to Kaplan-Meier analysis (log-rank, P = .83).

The 1- and 5-year overall survival rates for the subtotal resection group versus the subtotal resection plus radiotherapy group were 77% versus 88%, and 77% versus 17%, respectively. Although a trend was seen toward decreased overall survival in patients treated with subtotal resection plus radiotherapy, this difference was not statistically significant (log-rank, P = .14). These results suggest that postoperative adjuvant radiotherapy after subtotal resection does not significantly add to tumor control rates or survival compared with subtotal resection alone. Taken together with the inability of subtotal resection with radiotherapy to replace gross total resection, these results suggest that pineocytoma is a relative radioresistant lesion and, in the absence of better evidence suggesting radiotherapy is beneficial for this lesion, that conventional fractionated radiation treatment has a minimal role as either a sole or adjuvant treatment for pineocytoma. When evaluating a patient who has previously undergone a subtotal resection, repeat craniotomy with the goal of complete removal should be considered depending on surgeon comfort.

SUMMARY

Based on the rarity of pineocytoma and the long follow-up required to adequately document recurrence and overall survival, a prospective trial to address management issues is unlikely. In the absence of these data, current evidence indicates that surgical resection is the appropriate treatment for these tumors. When anatomically possible, gross total resection should be attempted, because this is associated with improved tumor control and longer progression-free and overall survivals. Adjuvant fractionated radiotherapy does not improve rate of tumor control or survival when used to treat a subtotally resected tumor. If possible, future studies are needed to address issues related to postoperative

neurovascular complications, particularly in patients who undergo gross total resection. Particular focus on preoperative variables such as tumor size, and operative technique such as patient position, will aid in surgical decision-making guidelines.

REFERENCES

1. Amendola BE, Wolf A, Coy SR, et al. Pineal tumors: analysis of treatment results in 20 patients. J Neurosurg 2005;102(Suppl):175–9.
2. Kida Y, Kobayashi T, Tanaka T, et al. Radiosurgery for bilateral neurinomas associated with neurofibromatosis type 2. Surg Neurol 2000;53:383–9 [discussion: 389–90].
3. Linskey ME, Lunsford LD, Flickinger JC. Radiosurgery for acoustic neurinomas: early experience. Neurosurgery 1990;26:736–44 [discussion: 744–5].
4. Deshmukh VR, Smith KA, Rekate HL, et al. Diagnosis and management of pineocytomas. Neurosurgery 2004;55:349–55 [discussion: 355–7].
5. Hasegawa T, Kondziolka D, Hadjipanayis CG, et al. The role of radiosurgery for the treatment of pineal parenchymal tumors. Neurosurgery 2002;51:880–9.
6. Jackson AS, Plowman PN. Pineal parenchymal tumours: I. Pineocytoma: a tumour responsive to platinum-based chemotherapy. Clin Oncol (R Coll Radiol) 2004;16:238–43.
7. Sakoda K, Uozumi T, Kawamoto K, et al. Responses of pineocytoma to radiation therapy and chemotherapy–report of two cases. Neurol Med Chir (Tokyo) 1989;29:825–9.
8. Clark AJ, Ivan ME, Sughrue ME, et al. Tumor control after surgery and radiotherapy for pineocytoma. J Neurosurg 2010;113:319–24.
9. Clark AJ, Sughrue ME, Ivan ME, et al. Factors influencing overall survival rates for patients with pineocytoma. J Neurooncol 2010;100:255–60.
10. Case records of the Massachusetts General Hospital. Weekly clinicopathological exercises. Case 35-1983. A 25-year-old woman with increasingly frequent headaches. N Engl J Med 1983;309:542–9.
11. Apuzzo ML, Stieg PE, Starr P, et al. Surgery of the Soul's cistern. Neurosurgery 1996;39:1022–9.
12. Barber SG, Smith JA, Hughes RC. Melatonin as a tumour marker in a patient with pineal tumour. Br Med J 1978;2:328.
13. Bendersky M, Lewis M, Mandelbaum DE, et al. Serial neuropsychological follow-up of a child following craniospinal irradiation. Dev Med Child Neurol 1988;30:816–20.
14. Borit A, Blackwood W, Mair WG. The separation of pineocytoma from pineoblastoma. Cancer 1980;45:1408–18.
15. D'Andrea AD, Packer RJ, Rorke LB, et al. Pineocytomas of childhood. A reappraisal of natural history and response to therapy. Cancer 1987;59:1353–7.

16. Dario A, Cerati M, Taborelli M, et al. Cytogenetic and ultrastructural study of a pineocytoma case report. J Neurooncol 2000;48:131–4.

17. Dempsey PK, Kondziolka D, Lunsford LD. Stereotactic diagnosis and treatment of pineal region tumours and vascular malformations. Acta Neurochir (Wien) 1992;116:14–22.

18. Disclafani A, Hudgins RJ, Edwards MS, et al. Pineocytomas. Cancer 1989;63:302–4.

19. Engel U, Gottschalk S, Niehaus L, et al. Cystic lesions of the pineal region—MRI and pathology. Neuroradiology 2000;42:399–402.

20. Fukushima T, Tomonaga M, Sawada T, et al. Pineocytoma with neuronal differentiation—case report. Neurol Med Chir (Tokyo) 1990;30:63–8.

21. Glanzmann C, Seelentag W. Radiotherapy for tumours of the pineal region and suprasellar germinomas. Radiother Oncol 1989;16:31–40.

22. Harada K, Hayashi T, Anegawa S, et al. Pineocytoma with intratumoral hemorrhage following ventriculoperitoneal shunt—case report. Neurol Med Chir (Tokyo) 1993;33:836–8.

23. Hazen S, Freiberg SR, Thomas C, et al. Multiple distinct intracranial tumors: association of pinealoma and craniopharyngioma. Case report. Surg Neurol 1989;31:381–6.

24. Herrick MK, Rubinstein LJ. The cytological differentiating potential of pineal parenchymal neoplasms (true pinealomas). A clinicopathological study of 28 tumours. Brain 1979;102:289–320.

25. Jooma R, Kendall BE. Diagnosis and management of pineal tumors. J Neurosurg 1983;58:654–65.

26. Jouvet A, Saint-Pierre G, Fauchon F, et al. Pineal parenchymal tumors: a correlation of histological features with prognosis in 66 cases. Brain Pathol 2000; 10:49–60.

27. Knierim DS, Yamada S. Pineal tumors and associated lesions: the effect of ethnicity on tumor type and treatment. Pediatr Neurosurg 2003;38:307–23.

28. Kobayashi T, Kida Y, Mori Y. Stereotactic gamma radiosurgery for pineal and related tumors. J Neurooncol 2001;54:301–9.

29. Koide O, Watanabe Y, Sato K. Pathological survey of intracranial germinoma and pinealoma in Japan. Cancer 1980;45:2119–30.

30. Kurisaka M, Arisawa M, Mori T, et al. Combination chemotherapy (cisplatin, vinblastin) and low-dose irradiation in the treatment of pineal parenchymal cell tumors. Childs Nerv Syst 1998;14:564–9.

31. Lee MA, Leng ME, Tiernan EJ. Risperidone: a useful adjunct for behavioural disturbance in primary cerebral tumours. Palliat Med 2001;15:255–6.

32. Linggood RM, Chapman PH. Pineal tumors. J Neurooncol 1992;12:85–91.

33. Mandera M, Marcol W, Bierzynska-Macyszyn G, et al. Pineal cysts in childhood. Childs Nerv Syst 2003;19:750–5.

34. Marcol W, Kotulska K, Grajkowska W, et al. Papillary pineocytoma in child: a case report. Biomed Pap Med Fac Univ Palacky Olomouc Czech Repub 2007;151:121–3.

35. Matsumoto K, Imaoka T, Tomita S, et al. Pineocytoma with massive intratumoral hemorrhage after ventriculoperitoneal shunt—case report. Neurol Med Chir (Tokyo) 1997;37:911–5.

36. Mawrin C, Grimm C, von Falkenhausen U, et al. Pineal epidermoid coinciding with pineocytoma. Acta Neurochir (Wien) 2003;145:783–7.

37. Mena H, Rushing EJ, Ribas JL, et al. Tumors of pineal parenchymal cells: a correlation of histological features, including nucleolar organizer regions, with survival in 35 cases. Hum Pathol 1995;26:20–30.

38. Miles A, Tidmarsh SF, Philbrick D, et al. Diagnostic potential of melatonin analysis in pineal tumors. N Engl J Med 1985;313:329–30.

39. Missori P, Delfini R, Cantore G. Tinnitus and hearing loss in pineal region tumours. Acta Neurochir (Wien) 1995;135:154–8.

40. Momozaki N, Ikezaki K, Abe M, et al. Cystic pineocytoma—case report. Neurol Med Chir (Tokyo) 1992; 32:169–71.

41. Munoz M, Page LK. Acquired double elevator palsy in a child with a pineocytoma. Am J Ophthalmol 1994;118:810–1.

42. Nakagawa H, Iwasaki S, Kichikawa K, et al. MR imaging of pineocytoma: report of two cases. AJNR Am J Neuroradiol 1990;11:195–8.

43. Nakamura M, Saeki N, Iwadate Y, et al. Neuroradiological characteristics of pineocytoma and pineoblastoma. Neuroradiology 2000;42:509–14.

44. Neuwelt EA. An update on the surgical treatment of malignant pineal region tumors. Clin Neurosurg 1985;32:397–428.

45. Neuwelt EA, Buchan C, Blank NK, et al. Surgical resection of a pineal tumor containing elements of germinoma and astrocytoma. Neurosurgery 1985; 16:373–8.

46. Neuwelt EA, Glasberg M, Frenkel E, et al. Malignant pineal region tumors. A clinico-pathological study. J Neurosurg 1979;51:597–607.

47. Packer RJ, Grossman RI, Rorke LB, et al. Brain stem necrosis after preradiation high-dose methotrexate. Childs Nerv Syst 1985;1:355–8.

48. Pople IK, Athanasiou TC, Sandeman DR, et al. The role of endoscopic biopsy and third ventriculostomy in the management of pineal region tumours. Br J Neurosurg 2001;15:305–11.

49. Prahlow JA, Challa VR. Neoplasms of the pineal region. South Med J 1996;89:1081–7.

50. Rainho CA, Rogatto SR, de Moraes LC, et al. Cytogenetic study of a pineocytoma. Cancer Genet Cytogenet 1992;64:127–32.

51. Reyns N, Hayashi M, Chinot O, et al. The role of Gamma Knife radiosurgery in the treatment of pineal

parenchymal tumours. Acta Neurochir (Wien) 2006; 148:5–11 [discussion: 11].

52. Rubinstein LJ, Okazaki H. Gangliogliomatous differentiation in a pineocytoma. J Pathol 1970;102:27–32.

53. Schulder M, Liang D, Carmel PW. Cranial surgery navigation aided by a compact intraoperative magnetic resonance imager. J Neurosurg 2001;94:936–45.

54. Schulte FJ, Herrmann HD, Muller D, et al. Pineal region tumours of childhood. Eur J Pediatr 1987; 146:233–45.

55. Shin E, Kim H, Kim TS, et al. Pleomorphic variant of pineocytoma—a case report. Korean J Pathol 2004; 38:265–7.

56. Shirane R, Shamoto H, Umezawa K, et al. Surgical treatment of pineal region tumours through the occipital transtentorial approach: evaluation of the effectiveness of intra-operative micro-endoscopy combined with neuronavigation. Acta Neurochir (Wien) 1999;141:801–8 [discussion: 808–9].

57. Steinbok P, Dolman CL, Kaan K. Pineocytomas presenting as subarachnoid hemorrhage. Report of two cases. J Neurosurg 1977;47:776–80.

58. Tamaki N, Yin D. Therapeutic strategies and surgical results for pineal region tumours. J Clin Neurosci 2000;7:125–8.

59. Tracy PT, Hanigan WC, Kalyan-Raman UP. Radiological and pathological findings in three cases of childhood pineocytomas. Childs Nerv Syst 1986;2:297–300.

60. Trojanowski JQ, Tascos NA, Rorke LB. Malignant pineocytoma with prominent papillary features. Cancer 1982;50:1789–93.

61. Tucker WG, Leong AS, McCulloch GA. Tumours of the pineal region—neuroradiological aspects. Australas Radiol 1977;21:313–24.

62. Ueki K, Tanaka R. Treatments and prognoses of pineal tumors—experience of 110 cases. Neurol Med Chir (Tokyo) 1980;20:1–26.

63. Vaquero J, Coca S, Martinez R, et al. Papillary pineocytoma. Case report. J Neurosurg 1990;73:135–7.

64. Vaquero J, Ramiro J, Martinez R, et al. Clinicopathological experience with pineocytomas: report of five surgically treated cases. Neurosurgery 1990;27: 612–8 [discussion: 618–9].

65. Vorkapic P, Pendl G. Microsurgery of pineal region lesions in children. Neuropediatrics 1987; 18:222–6.

66. Vorkapic P, Waldhauser F, Bruckner R, et al. Serum melatonin levels: a new neurodiagnostic tool in pineal region tumors? Neurosurgery 1987;21:817–24.

67. Weisberg LA. Clinical and computed tomographic correlations of pineal neoplasms. Comput Radiol 1984;8:285–92.

68. Ziyal IM, Sekhar LN, Salas E, et al. Combined supra/infratentorial-transsinus approach to large pineal region tumors. J Neurosurg 1998;88:1050–7.

69. Bruce JN, Ogden AT. Surgical strategies for treating patients with pineal region tumors. J Neurooncol 2004;69:221–36.

70. Kraichoke S, Cosgrove M, Chandrasoma PT. Granulomatous inflammation in pineal germinoma. A cause of diagnostic failure at stereotaxic brain biopsy. Am J Surg Pathol 1988;12:655–60.

71. Chaynes P. Microsurgical anatomy of the great cerebral vein of Galen and its tributaries. J Neurosurg 2003;99:1028–38.

72. Youssef AS, Downes AE, Agazzi S, et al. Life without the vein of Galen: clinical and radiographic sequelae. Clin Anat, in press. DOI:10.1002/ca.21176.

73. Lekovic GP, Gonzalez LF, Shetter AG, et al. Role of Gamma Knife surgery in the management of pineal region tumors. Neurosurg Focus 2007;23:E12.

74. Dandy WE. Operative experience in cases of pineal tumor. Arch Surg 1936;33:19–46.

75. Stoiber EM, Schaible B, Herfarth K, et al. Long term outcome of adolescent and adult patients with pineal parenchymal tumors treated with fractionated radiotherapy between 1982 and 2003—a single institution's experience. Radiat Oncol 2010;5:122.

Contemporary Management of Pineoblastoma

Matthew C. Tate, MD, PhD, Martin J. Rutkowski, BA,
Andrew T. Parsa, MD, PhD*

KEYWORDS

• Pineoblastoma • Survival • Treatment

Pineal tumors comprise 1% of all primary central nervous system (CNS) neoplasms. Germ cell tumors (GCTs) are the most common pineal tumors (35%), followed by pineal parenchymal tumors (PPTs, 30%). Other less common pineal region tumors include astrocytomas and ependymomas.[1] A new class of tumors termed papillary pineal tumors was introduced by the World Health Organization (WHO) in 2007.[2] Among the PPTs, there are 3 major subgroups: pineocytoma (WHO grade I), PPTs of intermediate differentiation (WHO grade II/III), and pineoblastoma (PB) (WHO grade IV).

PBs comprise 25% to 50% of PPTs and are most commonly seen in children and adolescents, with an average age at diagnosis of 13 years.[3–5] These tumors are considered primary neuroectodermal tumors (PNETs) of the pineal region and exhibit aggressive clinical behavior with frequent metastases throughout the craniospinal axis.[6,7] Histologic analysis of PBs reveals hypercellularity, high nuclear-to-cytoplasm ratio, and frequent mitoses (17%–40%).[8] Homer-Wright or Flexner-Wintersteiner rosettes may also be present (**Fig. 1**). Immunohistochemical markers characteristic of PB include synaptophysin and neuron-specific enolase, along with variable staining for glial fibrillary acidic protein, chromogranin A, and neurofilaments.[1] Recent genetic analyses of PB demonstrate several upregulated genes (UBEC2, SOX4, TERT, TEP1, PRAME, CD24, POU4F2, HOXD13) and chromosomal abnormalities (1p rearrangement, 22q loss).[8,9] Standard of care in the United States includes maximal surgical resection with adjuvant craniospinal irradiation and systemic chemotherapy,[10] resulting in a median survival of 16 to 25 months[5] and a 5-year survival rate of 10%.[3] This review discusses the principles of contemporary management of PB.

CLINICAL PRESENTATION AND INITIAL MANAGEMENT

Patients with PB most commonly present with findings of elevated intracranial pressure (ICP) (headache, nausea/vomiting, and decreased level of consciousness) as a result of obstructive hydrocephalus from compression of the cerebral aqueduct by the tumor mass. Patients may also exhibit Parinaud syndrome (upgaze paralysis, convergence nystagmus, and near-light dissociation) as a result of compression of the dorsal midbrain structures. Focal neurologic deficits are present in approximately 25% of patients and are found incidentally in 5%.[7]

Initial workup includes a careful neurologic history and physical examination, including a fundoscopic examination. In particular, the presence or absence of focal neurologic deficits, altered level of consciousness, papilledema, and extraocular movement abnormalities are noted. If a significant level of suspicion is present, the next step is intracranial imaging, typically brain magnetic resonance imaging (MRI) with and without contrast. Key features are the characteristics of the pineal mass (size, enhancement pattern, and solid vs cystic) as well as the presence and degree of

Disclosure: The authors have no financial interests or conflicts of interest to disclose.
Department of Neurological Surgery, University of California, San Francisco, 505 Parnassus Avenue, M779, Box 0112, San Francisco, CA 94117, USA
* Corresponding author.
E-mail address: parsaa@neurosurg.ucsf.edu

Neurosurg Clin N Am 22 (2011) 409–412
doi:10.1016/j.nec.2011.05.001
1042-3680/11/$ /$ – see front matter © 2011 Published by Elsevier Inc.

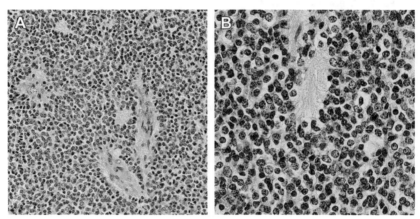

Fig. 1. Histopathology of PB demonstrating classic hypercellularity of small undifferentiated cells with delicate, blunt cytoplasmic processes (*A*) (hematoxylin-eosin, original magnification ×50) and Homer-Wright rosettes (*B*) (hematoxylin-eosin, original magnification ×100).

obstructive hydrocephalus (**Fig. 2**). Patients with signs of elevated ICP (papilledema, decreased visual acuity) and obstructive hydrocephalus should be admitted for urgent cerebrospinal fluid (CSF) diversion (see the section on Hydrocephalus treatment and CSF sampling). An important distinction among pineal masses is that of a pineal cyst, which is a common benign lesion isointense to CSF. These lesions can be followed with serial MRI scans and in most cases do not require further intervention. Given the propensity of some pineal tumors to metastasize to the spinal column (PB, ependymoma, or germinoma), a baseline contrast-enhanced MRI of the entire spinal axis should be obtained. In addition to further imaging, the presence of a pineal tumor should also prompt sampling of GCT markers (β-human chorionic gonadotropin or α-fetoprotein) from serum and/or CSF. Most commonly, CSF is obtained during the initial CSF diversion procedure (see the section on Hydrocephalus treatment and CSF sampling) and sent for GCT markers and cytology.

HYDROCEPHALUS TREATMENT AND CSF SAMPLING

Given that most patients with pineal tumors present with symptoms related to hydrocephalus, a common first procedure is an endoscopic third ventriculostomy (ETV) or ventriculoperitoneal shunt. Either procedure allows for both CSF sampling (important for ruling out GCTs as discussed above) and alleviation of obstructive hydrocephalus, which is the most pressing concern during acute management of patients with PB. Patients with CSF positive for GCT markers should then receive adjuvant therapy without the need for further surgical intervention.

Among the CSF diversion options, most neurosurgeons prefer ETV because it offers permanent relief of hydrocephalus without indwelling hardware and the possibility of an endoscopic biopsy during the same surgical procedure.

SURGICAL MANAGEMENT

After treatment of obstructive hydrocephalus and confirming negative CSF markers/cytology, the next step in the management of PB is establishing a tissue diagnosis. Options include stereotactic biopsy, endoscopic biopsy, or open surgery. Stereotactic biopsy of pineal masses is associated with a higher degree of hemorrhage relative to biopsy of other CNS sites,[11] although the clinical significance of this increased rate is not well established.[12] Another minimally invasive approach is an endoscopic biopsy, which has the advantage of being able to be performed at the time of ETV. However, when using a traditional rigid endoscope, this requires a second burr hole, because a lower trajectory than that used for the ETV is needed for accessing the pineal region. It is also possible to use a flexible endoscope through the original ETV burr hole. A major disadvantage of endoscopic biopsy via either approach is the difficulty in controlling intraventricular bleeding at the biopsy site. Irrespective of the method used, biopsies only sample a small portion of the tumor and may result in a missed or inaccurate diagnosis in approximately 10% of cases.[13] For these reasons, the treatment of choice for most PPTs, including PB, remains open surgical resection. Open surgery allows for adequate tissue sampling and improved diagnostic accuracy, which is critical for effective management of pineal lesions. In addition, aggressive surgical resection is associated

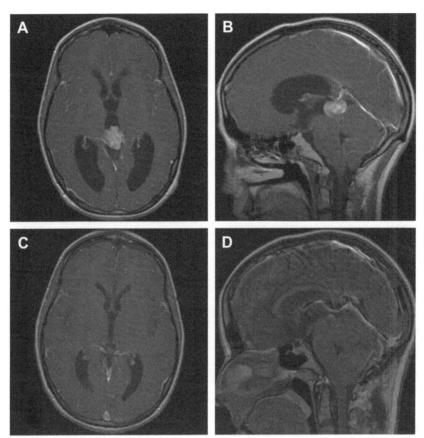

Fig. 2. Preoperative (A, B) and postoperative (C, D) T1-weighted, gadolinium-enhanced brain magnetic resonance images of a patient with tissue-confirmed PB. Axial (A) and sagittal (B) images demonstrate a mass with obstructive hydrocephalus in the pineal region. Surgery was performed via a supracerebellar infratentorial approach with the patient in the sitting position, resulting in a gross total resection as observed on the axial (C) and sagittal (D) images.

with improved outcome in both pineocytoma (gross total resection is often curative, obviating the need for adjuvant therapy) and PB (gross total resection results in prolonged survival). Specific approaches to the pineal region are reviewed elsewhere in this issue, but the most common is the supracerebellar infratentorial approach, which is ideal for separating tumor from the deep venous system safely. Other common approaches include interhemispheric transcallosal and occipital transtentorial approaches. The rate of major perioperative surgical morbidity and mortality in recent series is 0% to 5%,[14,15] supporting an aggressive role for neurosurgeons in resecting PPTs.

ADJUVANT THERAPY

Standard adjuvant therapy for pathology-confirmed PB after maximal surgical resection includes fractionated radiotherapy and chemotherapy. Typical radiotherapy protocols for PB are 5500 cGy to the tumor region and 3500 cGy to the spinal axis

(2 Gy fractions). Chemotherapy protocols are less consistent among centers but usually include 2 to 3 agents selected from vincristine, cisplatin/carboplatin, cyclophosphamide, etoposide, and CCNU (lomustine).[10,16] In addition to these standard therapies, more recent modalities such as Gamma Knife radiotherapy have been suggested as an adjunct to conventional radiotherapy or as a substitute for surgical resection,[17] but definitive data are lacking. Several promising experimental therapies are being evaluated for the treatment of PB, including vorinostat (a histone deacetylase inhibitor), retinoic acid, and high-dose chemotherapy with autologous stem cell rescue.[10,18]

OUTCOMES

Survival rates for patients with PB remain poor, with a median survival of 20 months and a 5-year survival rate of 10%.[3,5] Patient factors that have consistently and independently predicted improved survival rate are (1) increased age at presentation (older than 3 years), (2) gross total resection (vs subtotal or biopsy), (3) lack of disseminated disease, and (4) craniospinal radiotherapy more than 40 Gy.[7,19] In addition to improved survival, craniospinal radiotherapy has also been shown to improve functional status,[7] suggesting a role in improving quality of life and survival. A recent study by Gilheeney and colleagues[10] also suggests a survival benefit for chemotherapy given in addition to radiotherapy and surgical resection.

SUMMARY

PBs represent the most aggressive of the PPTs. Routine treatment consists of operative management of obstructive hydrocephalus and CSF studies followed by maximal resection and adjuvant chemotherapy/radiotherapy, resulting in a median survival of 20 months. Important prognostic factors for survival of patients with PB include the extent of resection, age at presentation, disseminated disease, and craniospinal radiotherapy. Novel strategies being evaluated for the treatment of PB include high-dose chemotherapy with autologous stem cell therapy, stereotactic radiosurgery, and histone deacetylase inhibitors.

REFERENCES

1. Dahiya S, Perry A. Pineal tumors. Adv Anat Pathol 2010;17:419–27.
2. Louis DN, Ohgaki H, Wiestler OD, et al. Tumors of the pineal region. In: Louis DN, Ohgaki H, Wiestler OD, et al, editors. WHO classification of tumors of the central nervous system. Geneva (Switzerland): WHO Press; 2007. p. 8.
3. Fauchon F, Jouvet A, Paquis P, et al. Parenchymal pineal tumors: a clinicopathological study of 76 cases. Int J Radiat Oncol Biol Phys 2000;46:959–68.
4. Hart MN, Earle KM. Primitive neuroectodermal tumors of the brain in children. Cancer 1973;32:890–7.
5. Mena H, Rushing EJ, Ribas JL, et al. Tumors of pineal parenchymal cells: a correlation of histological features, including nucleolar organizer regions, with survival in 35 cases. Hum Pathol 1995;26:20–30.
6. Chang SM, Lillis-Hearne PK, Larson DA, et al. Pineoblastoma in adults. Neurosurgery 1995;37:383–90 [discussion: 390–1].
7. Lee JY, Wakabayashi T, Yoshida J. Management and survival of pineoblastoma: an analysis of 34 adults from the brain tumor registry of Japan. Neurol Med Chir (Tokyo) 2005;45:132–41 [discussion: 141–2].
8. Rickert CH, Simon R, Bergmann M, et al. Comparative genomic hybridization in pineal parenchymal tumors. Genes Chromosomes Cancer 2001;30:99–104.
9. Fevre-Montange M, Champier J, Szathmari A, et al. Microarray analysis reveals differential gene expression patterns in tumors of the pineal region. J Neuropathol Exp Neurol 2006;65:675–84.
10. Gilheeney SW, Saad A, Chi S, et al. Outcome of pediatric pineoblastoma after surgery, radiation and chemotherapy. J Neurooncol 2008;89:89–95.
11. Field M, Witham TF, Flickinger JC, et al. Comprehensive assessment of hemorrhage risks and outcomes after stereotactic brain biopsy. J Neurosurg 2001;94:545–51.
12. Regis J, Bouillot P, Rouby-Volot F, et al. Pineal region tumors and the role of stereotactic biopsy: review of the mortality, morbidity, and diagnostic rates in 370 cases. Neurosurgery 1996;39:907–12 [discussion: 912–4].
13. Konovalov AN, Pitskhelauri DI. Principles of treatment of the pineal region tumors. Surg Neurol 2003;59:250–68.
14. Bruce JN, Stein BM. Surgical management of pineal region tumors. Acta Neurochir (Wien) 1995;134:130–5.
15. Shin HJ, Cho BK, Jung HW, et al. Pediatric pineal tumors: need for a direct surgical approach and complications of the occipital transtentorial approach. Childs Nerv Syst 1998;14:174–8.
16. Tate MC, Banerjee A, Vandenberg SR, et al. Postradiation reactive changes in a single vertebral body mimicking metastatic pineoblastoma. J Neurosurg Pediatr 2009;4:479–83.
17. Lekovic GP, Gonzalez LF, Shetter AG, et al. Role of Gamma Knife surgery in the management of pineal region tumors. Neurosurg Focus 2007;23:E12.
18. DeBoer R, Batjer H, Marymont M, et al. Response of an adult patient with pineoblastoma to vorinostat and retinoic acid. J Neurooncol 2009;95:289–92.
19. Stoiber EM, Schaible B, Herfarth K, et al. Long term outcome of adolescent and adult patients with pineal parenchymal tumors treated with fractionated radiotherapy between 1982 and 2003—a single institution's experience. Radiat Oncol 2010;5:122.

Stereotactic Radiosurgery for Pineal Region Tumors

Simon J. Hanft, MD*, Steven R. Isaacson, MD,
Jeffrey N. Bruce, MD

KEYWORDS

- Stereotactic radiosurgery • Pineal region tumors
- Microsurgery

The role of radiosurgery in the management of pineal region tumors is still in its incipient stages, although over the past few years its use has expanded, both as a primary treatment modality and as an adjunct to conventional therapies. Because of the rarity of pineal region tumors, which account for 0.4% to 1% of all adult intracranial tumors in the United States and Europe (3%–8% in children), there are no clearly defined criteria for the use of radiosurgery, and controversy still exists regarding the best use of this intervention.[1] Although there have been advances in microsurgical approaches that have significantly reduced the morbidity of open surgical procedures, resection of pineal region tumors remains challenging and brings with it the potential of adverse effects.[2] The combined risk of morbidity and mortality of these open approaches has ranged from 30% to 70% in the older literature,[3] prompting a period when empirical fractionated radiation therapy was occasionally used as a first-line treatment.[4] The advent of stereotactic radiosurgery, therefore, presented a noninvasive alternative modality that has subsequently gained traction among neurosurgeons and neuro-oncologists in recent years.

Looking back over the past decade, there have been several retrospective clinical studies that have begun to establish the efficacy and safety of radiosurgery for pineal region tumors, despite the histologic diversity presented by tumors in this anatomic location. The stereotactic radiosurgical modality of choice has been Gamma Knife radiosurgery (GKRS), although there are some earlier reports of linear accelerator (LINAC) radiosurgery of pineal region tumors.[5] There are no published reports of CyberKnife radiosurgery to tumors of the pineal region. The goal of this article is to give a detailed overview of the recent literature regarding the merits of stereotactic radiosurgery to pineal region tumors, and to offer the practicing neurosurgeon and neuro-oncologist reasonable guidelines for the incorporation of radiosurgery into the clinical management of these difficult lesions.

STEREOTACTIC RADIOSURGERY: WHICH TUMORS ARE BEST?

It is currently recommended that patients with pineal region tumors carry a diagnosis before the initiation of radiosurgery. Given the wide range of histologic varieties present in this region, determination of tumor type has a significant impact on clinical management. Typically, tissue diagnosis is obtained via stereotactic biopsy, and often this surgical procedure is supplemented by markers found in the serum and cerebrospinal fluid (CSF) (α-fetoprotein [AFP], human chorionic gonadotropin [β-HCG], carcinoembryonic antigen, placental alkaline phosphatase). In general, stereotactic radiosurgery has been advocated for radiosensitive malignant pineal region tumors as well as for local control of benign tumors.[5] There has also been an increasing trend toward using radiosurgery for postoperative residual tumor.[3] The three broad categories of tumor treated by stereotactic radiosurgery include pineal parenchymal tumors (PPTs, which include both pineocytomas and

Department of Neurological Surgery, Columbia University College of Physicians and Surgeons, Room 434, Neurological Institute, Columbia University Medical Center, 710 West 168th Street, New York, NY 10032, USA
* Corresponding author.
E-mail address: sihanft@gmail.com

Neurosurg Clin N Am 22 (2011) 413–420
doi:10.1016/j.nec.2011.05.002
1042-3680/11/$ – see front matter © 2011 Elsevier Inc. All rights reserved.

pineoblastomas), germ cell tumors (GCTs) (germinomatous and nongerminomatous [NGGCTs]), and glial tumors (astrocytomas). Beginning with PPTs, the remainder of this article discusses the indications, efficacy, safety, and outcomes of stereotactic radiosurgery on each tumor subtype within these broad categories.

PPTs
Pineocytoma

PPTs comprise from 15% to 30% of all pineal region tumors, and pineocytomas make up about 30% to 60% of PPTs.[6] The category of PPTs includes pineocytomas, mixed pineocytomas/pineoblastomas (PPTs of intermediate differentiation [PPTID]), and pineoblastomas. Pineocytomas are slow-growing tumors that arise from the parenchyma of the pineal gland and are classified as World Health Organization (WHO) grade II lesions. As is the case with many tumor types arising within the pineal region, pineocytomas are rare lesions and remain underrepresented in the literature in terms of receiving stereotactic radiosurgery.

A recent large retrospective study by Mori and colleagues[7] examined the safety and efficacy of GKRS (KULA system, Elekta, Tokyo) as an adjuvant treatment on 49 patients with 74 tumors involving the pineal region over a 15-year period. Specifically, 9 patients presented with PPTs (19 tumors in total), and all PPTs were diagnosed by histologic confirmation. Furthermore, all PPT cases underwent surgical resection before GKRS, making the radiosurgical intervention in this study a postoperative, adjuvant modality. Thirteen total pineocytomas found in 6 patients were included in the study. The marginal dose of GKRS ranged from 12.5 to 20.3 Gy and the maximum dose ranged from 17 to 40 Gy (Table 1); these doses include all PPTs and the investigators do not designate the radiation values for pineocytomas only. In addition, the local tumor control (LTC) rate at 3 and 5 years was 85%, and the progression-free survival (PFS) rate at 3 and 5

years was 80%. These were the highest LTC and PFS rates in the study, leading the investigators to conclude that GKRS is both safe and effective as an adjuvant treatment of pineocytomas.

Kano and colleagues[8] simultaneously published their institutional experience with pineocytomas over a 20-year period. All PPTs in this study were histologically confirmed; 6 of the 20 patients studied had previous surgical resection, and of these 6 patients, 3 underwent previous fractionated radiation therapy, 3 received chemotherapy, and 2 received both. The investigators do not specify which histologic type underwent surgery initially and/or adjuvant therapy before the initiation of GKRS (Elekta Inc, Atlanta, GA, USA). This study included 13 patients with pineocytomas; the margin dose of GKRS ranged from 12 to 20 Gy, whereas the maximum dose ranged from 24 to 40 Gy (see Table 1). No instances of progressive disease were noted among the patients with pineocytoma; 3 patients experienced a complete response, 8 patients showed a partial response, and 2 patients had evidence of stable disease. The survival rates and PFS rates were also remarkably high in this patient group: actuarial 1-year, 3-year, and 5-year survival rates were 100%, 92.3%, and 92.3%, respectively. PFS rates were 100% at 1, 3, and 5 years. The conclusion drawn from this study regarding GKRS treatment of pineocytomas, therefore, was that stereotactic radiosurgery is both a safe and effective alternative to open surgical resection.

Lekovic and colleagues[9] include 8 patients with pineocytoma in their retrospective analysis of GKRS (Leksell GammaPlan, Elekta, Tokyo) for pineal region tumors. All of these patients underwent biopsy leading to a tissue diagnosis before institution of GKRS. The peak dose ranged from 26 to 32 Gy. Among these 8 patients, half showed a partial response, whereas the other half showed no change in symptoms (see Table 1). Despite the high rates of tumor control that these investigators reported, they still concluded that craniotomy

---

Table 1
A study-by-study summary of GKRS in the treatment of pineocytomas

Investigators	Number of Tumors	Tumor Volume: Range, Mean (mL)	Marginal Dose: Range, Mean (Gy)	Maximum Dose: Range, Mean (Gy)	PFS at 3 and 5 y (%)
Mori et al[7]	13	0.3–23.0, 3.7	12.5–20.3, 16.7	17.0–40.0, 27.9	80; 80
Kano et al[8]	13	0.9–14.2, 4.4	12–20, 15.2	24–40, 30.4	100; 100
Lekovic et al[9]	8	1.9–12.4, 6.0	N/A	26–32, 28.8	N/A
Deshmukh et al[11]	5	1.9–9.6, 6.4	14–16, 14.8	N/A	N/A
Reyns et al[3]	8	N/A	N/A	24–40, 30.2	N/A

Abbreviation: N/A, not applicable.

with an attempt at gross total resection (GTR) is the best treatment approach for benign tumors such as pineocytomas given that this is the closest guarantee to a definitive cure. However, the investigators did state that based on their data, GKRS has potential as a primary treatment modality for pineocytomas, especially in cases in which GTR is deemed impossible or achievable only at an unacceptable risk to the patient. In the final analysis, the Lekovic study supported surgery with an attempt at GTR over GKRS as the primary intervention, with GKRS reserved for treatment of residual or recurrent disease or in cases in which GTR comes at too high a cost. More recent literature supports this conclusion, namely a study by Clark and colleagues[10] that examined the benefits of GTR versus subtotal resection (STR) combined with adjuvant radiation therapy. This study concluded that GTR leads to tumor control rates suggestive of a complete cure compared with STR and radiotherapy. Moreover, STR alone versus STR and radiotherapy showed no difference in tumor control rates, suggesting that postoperative adjuvant radiotherapy offers no advantage in the treatment of subtotally resected lesions. The investigators note in this review that the postoperative radiotherapy in their retrospective patient population is either fractionated radiotherapy or stereotactic radiosurgery, but there is no subgroup analysis involving the patients who received stereotactic radiosurgery. Therefore, it is difficult to extend these investigators' conclusion to include all patients undergoing stereotactic radiosurgery, as well as those patients who undergo stereotactic radiosurgery as a primary treatment modality. Before this study, Deshmukh and colleagues[11] arrived at a similar conclusion regarding pineocytomas, albeit within a smaller sample size (9 patients compared with 166 patients in the study by Clark and colleagues). Within this small sample, only 5 patients underwent GKRS, but all showed either LTC or reduction of tumor size. The investigators therefore concluded that radiosurgery seems to be effective for LTC, despite the small sample size and short follow-up period (19.3 months).

The retrospective study from Reyns and colleagues[3] included 8 patients with pineocytomas; 6 of these patients were treated primarily with GKRS (Leksell Gamma Knife models B and C, Elekta, Tokyo), whereas the other 2 underwent GKRS after subtotal surgical resection. The central dose ranged from 24 to 40 Gy. Of the 6 patients undergoing GKRS as a primary intervention, 1 patient showed complete regression, 3 patients showed partial regression of at least 50%, and 2 patients had no change in the size of the tumor (see **Table 1**). Of the 2 patients who underwent

GKRS after STR, one was lost to follow-up, whereas the other patient showed partial regression. The investigators conclude from these data that GKRS is an effective primary treatment modality in the case of pineocytomas and can serve as the sole means of intervention in such patients.

Pineoblastoma

Pineoblastomas are highly malignant parenchymal tumors of the pineal region that account for approximately 4% of PPTs and are classified as WHO Grade IV lesions.[12] These tumors realize their malignant potential in the form of CSF seeding (14%–43% of cases) as well as extracranial metastases (most commonly bone).[1] Mean survival time after multimodal intervention (surgery, chemotherapy, radiation) is typically around 2 years; overall 5-year survival ranges from 10% to 51%, and without treatment survival may be only a few months.[12,13] Similar to their benign PPT counterpart, the pineocytoma, pineoblastomas are exceedingly rare lesions and there is limited experience treating these lesions with stereotactic radiosurgery.

Mori and colleagues[7] include only 4 pineoblastomas (2 patients) in their large retrospective study of 49 patients, illustrating the scarcity of this tumor type. As noted earlier, the study combined pineoblastomas, pineocytomas, and PPTIDs (referred to as mixed pineocytoma/pineoblastoma in this article) in their GKRS dose planning data, so the 4 pineoblastomas fall within the treatment ranges mentioned earlier. Given that there was only 1 patient with a PPTID, the investigators combined this patient with the 4 pineoblastomas in the data analysis. Significantly, the LTC rate for this group was only 30% at 2 years, whereas the PFS rate at 2 years was 33% (**Table 2**). There was a statistically significant difference in LTC between the pineocytoma group and the pineoblastoma/PPTID group, while the difference in PFS approached statistical significance. Both pineoblastoma patients in this study had evidence of tumor progression at 3 and 13 months after GKRS. Based on these data, especially because the pineoblastomas both relapsed, the investigators do not recommend GKRS as an adjuvant therapy in the management of pineoblastoma.

Of the 20 patients with PPT analyzed in the Kano and colleagues[8] study, 5 patients had pineoblastomas and 2 patients had mixed tumors (PPTID). The GKRS dosing plan mentioned earlier in the setting of the pineocytomas reported in this study includes the pineoblastomas and PPTIDs as well. Based on follow-up imaging, there were 2 pineoblastomas with complete tumor resolution, 1

Table 2
Breakdown of pineoblastoma treatment parameters including PFS

Investigators	Number of Tumors	Tumor Volume: Range, Mean (mL)	Marginal Dose: Range, Mean (Gy)	Maximum Dose: Range, Mean (Gy)	PFS at 3 and 5 y (%)
Mori et al[7]	4	0.3–23.0, 3.7	12.5–20.3, 16.7	17.0–40.0, 27.9	33 (2 yrs)
Kano et al[8]	5	0.9–14.2, 4.4	12–20, 15.2	24–40, 30.4	66.7; 66.7
Lekovic et al[9]	1	23.0, 23.0	N/A	28, 28	100
Reyns et al[3]	5	N/A	N/A	28–50, 33.6	N/A

Abbreviation: N/A, not applicable.

tumor had tumor regression, and 1 tumor was unchanged. However, in 2 patients with pineoblastomas, tumor progression was noted at 12.8 and 31.2 months, leading to repeat GKRS in one of these patients. The actuarial survival rates and PFS rates were significantly lower in the patients with pineoblastoma compared with those with pineocytoma, in keeping with previous studies (see **Table 2**). In terms of overall survival, the 1-year, 3-year, and 5-year rates were 95%, 80%, and 68.6%, respectively. These numbers compare favorably with those quoted in the Schild and colleagues[6] study, in which patients underwent various treatments, leading the investigators to suggest that adjuvant GKRS as part of an aggressive oncologic intervention may improve outcomes for pineoblastomas. This finding prompted the investigators to conclude that GKRS can prove an important adjunct in the multimodal treatment of pineoblastomas.

One patient with pineoblastoma is included in the Lekovic and colleagues[9] study, with histologic confirmation coming from open biopsy. The maximum dose to this tumor was 28 Gy, and there was no change in tumor size on follow-up imaging at 45 months after GKRS (see **Table 2**). This was the second largest tumor of the 17 tumors included in the study (23.0 cm³). The investigators used GKRS as adjuvant therapy in this pineoblastoma, but it is unclear whether it was the sole adjuvant treatment or combined with conventional external beam radiation therapy (EBRT)/intensity modulated radiation therapy. Given that these investigators had only 1 pineoblastoma in their series, they understandably refrain from drawing any conclusions about the role of GKRS in its management.

The study by Reyns and colleagues[3] included a total of 5 pineoblastomas, most of which were subjected to different management protocols. GKRS was the initial intervention in 1 case of pineoblastoma; it followed STR in 1 case; it was instituted before chemotherapy in 1 case of recurrent pineoblastoma that was initially treated with surgery and radiation; and in another 2 cases, GKRS was performed as a sandwich protocol between 2 chemotherapy sessions.[3] The maximum dose ranged from 28 to 50 Gy; complete regression was observed in 2 patients, complete regression but with brain metastasis in 1 patient, partial regression (90%) in 1 patient, and progression in 1 patient (see **Table 2**). The patient with progression died 36 months after GKRS as a result of tumor size progression, whereas the patient with partial regression of 90% died 20 months after GKRS from carcinomatous meningitis. Based on these limited data, the investigators conclude that the combination of GKRS with chemotherapy is an effective management strategy to induce LTC. However, they cannot faithfully conclude that GKRS confers any control over leptomeningeal spread, and they state that aggressive chemotherapy and/or craniospinal irradiation are critical in reducing the risk of distant metastasis.

The fundamental conclusion from these studies is that GKRS alone seems ineffective in treating pineoblastomas but that in combination with adjuvant treatments it has shown potential for controlling local tumor growth and possibly improving overall survival. An early study by Manera and colleagues[14] is essentially the only such study that found stereotactic radiosurgery alone (LINAC radiosurgery, not GKRS, Leksell Gamma Knife model B [Elekta]) to be effective in treating pineoblastomas, albeit in 2 patients. Thus, the question remains as to the exact role of GKRS in the multimodal treatment of pineoblastomas: is it a substitute for conventional EBRT or simply an additional tool in the armamentarium of the neuro-oncologist?

GCTs
Germinomas

GCTs are the most frequently found tumors in the pineal region, accounting for 31% to 85% of all pineal region tumors. They are divided into germinomatous and NGGCT categories, with the former including germinomas and the latter including teratomas (both mature and immature), embryonal carcinoma, yolk sac tumors, and choriocarcinoma.[1] In general, germinomas are extremely radiosensitive, and as such have the best prognosis. Mature teratomas are also associated with a good prognosis if GTR is possible, whereas all other NGGCTs carry poor prognoses. Five-year survival rates in germinomas after radiotherapy alone can reach 90%.[15] In Japan, where germinomas are more common, combined chemotherapy and/or conventional EBRT have exceeded a 90% cure rate.[16] Given this success rate in treating germinomas, the role for GKRS seems to be in the setting of recurrent or resistant tumor. The literature on GKRS in treating pineal germinomas is limited and does not venture beyond the small retrospective case series discussed here.

The experience of Mori and colleagues[7] in treating pineal region germinomas with GKRS provides the largest case series to date. Of the 38 patients with GCTs (53 total tumors) in the study, 16 harbored germinomas (18 total tumors), 6 had germinomas with syncytiotrophoblastic giant cells (STGC, a more malignant form of germinoma), and only one of the germinomas underwent GKRS as an initial treatment. The maximum dose of GKRS to the germinomas ranged from 14.5 to 40 Gy, and the marginal dose ranged from 9.9 to 25.7 Gy (included in the GKRS dose planning data are the malignant GCTs, or NGGCTs, which the investigators did not separate when presenting these data). Rates of LTC for germinomas at 3 and 5 years were both 82%, whereas PFS rates at 3 and 5 years were 79% and 63% (**Table 3**). The investigators specifically point out that only 25% of germinomas had tumor progression after GKRS. However, in the 1 patient who received GKRS as an initial treatment, there was CSF dissemination 15 months later, leading the

investigators to state that GKRS may not be recommended as an initial treatment of germinoma. GKRS emerged as an effective and safe adjuvant treatment in the case of germinoma but not as an initial therapy.

A case report of 3 patients from Japan with germinomas examined the efficacy of GKRS as an adjuvant treatment. Endo and colleagues[17] reported that GKRS (Leksell GammaPlan, Elekta, Tokyo) to these 3 germinomas at a marginal dose of 10 to 12 Gy, followed by whole ventricular irradiation (24 Gy), led to a complete response in all 3 patients with no recurrence. These patients did not undergo biopsy; rather the diagnosis was based on clinical and radiographic features of the lesion, as is commonly practiced in Japan. The investigators recommend this unique combination radiotherapy for GKRS, with whole ventricular irradiation as an initial and definitive treatment of germinoma.

Two smaller and more distant studies used GKRS for pineal germinomas. Manera and colleagues[14] included 2 patients with germinomas who underwent GKRS (Leksell Gamma Knife model B, Elekta, Tokyo) as an initial and solitary treatment. There was complete disappearance of both tumors at 7 and 15 days, and no evidence of recurrence at 13 and 19 months. Subach and colleagues[18] reported similar success in 2 cases of germinoma, both of which underwent GKRS and decreased in size.

The significantly limited experience with GKRS as a treatment of pineal germinomas makes it difficult to draw any substantiated or broad conclusions. The high success rate and relatively low morbidity of current radiotherapy for pineal germinomas seem to relegate GKRS to the role of adjuvant treatment, although the scant data from the early studies referenced here suggest that GKRS may have an expanded role as a primary intervention. More studies are necessary to determine how GKRS should be used, if at all, in treating germinomas.

Table 3
Dosimetry and PFS in germinomas and NGGCTs undergoing GKRS

Investigators	Number of Tumors	Tumor Volume: Range, Mean (mL)	Marginal Dose: Range, Mean (Gy)	Maximum Dose: Range, Mean (Gy)	PFS at 3 and 5 y (%)
Mori et al[7] (GCT)	18	0.1–22.0, 3.3	9.9–25.7, 15.5	14.5–40.0, 27.4	79; 63
Mori et al[7] (NGGCT)	16	0.1–22.0, 3.3	9.9–25.7, 15.5	14.5–40.0, 27.4	43; 37
Endo et al[17] (GCT)	3	<3, N/A	10–12, 11.0	N/A	N/A
Lekovic et al[9]	2	1.2–2.1, 1.6	N/A	26–30, 28.0	N/A
Hasegawa et al[20]	4	2.2–23.4, 10.5	12–16, 14.0	24–32, 28.0	N/A

Abbreviation: N/A, not applicable.

NGGCTs

NGGCTs are associated with a worse prognosis compared with GCTs; including all tumor subtypes in this category, 5-year survival rates with aggressive therapy ranges from 9% to 49%.[1] Biopsy is often unnecessary with these lesions given their association with increased β-HCG or AFP levels, although these markers can be normal in some cases.[5] Although these tumors are significantly less radiosensitive than germinomas, radiotherapy is still a critical aspect of the multimodal treatment approach. Because of the difficulty in treating these lesions, there has been greater interest in establishing the efficacy of GKRS than in germinomas, which are responsive to conventional radiotherapy. The subtypes within the NGGCT category are exceedingly rare tumors of the pineal region, and few investigators report their experience treating these lesions with GKRS.

As was the case with germinomas, Mori and colleagues[7] report the largest case series to date involving NGGCTs and GKRS. Of the 38 patients with GCTs (53 total tumors), there were 16 patients with NGGCTs, which are defined in this study as malignant GCTs. Only one of these underwent GKRS as an initial treatment. In presenting the data on LTC and PFS, the investigators include germinomas with STGC as part of the malignant GCT group, making it difficult to determine the impact of GKRS on the NGGCT subtypes alone (as noted earlier, germinomas with STGC are a more malignant form of germinoma and are therefore not considered NGGCTs). The GKRS dose planning data are mentioned earlier (see also **Table 3**). LTC rates for this group at 3 and 5 years were 72% and 62%, whereas the rates of PFS at 3 and 5 years were 43% and 37% (see **Table 3**). The investigators note a statistically significant difference between the PFS rates of germinomas and the malignant GCTs. The most efficacious regimen in treating NGGCTs has been combined chemotherapy with conventional irradiation followed by so-called second-look surgery in the event of persistent disease on follow-up imaging and in the presence of normalized CSF markers.[5] Five-year survival rates approaching 90% have been achieved through this strategy.[19] In the Mori and colleagues study, high mortality followed GKRS (31%) during a median follow-up of 20 months with PFS in only 50% of the cases for a median of 65 months. The 1 patient treated with GKRS as an initial therapy developed distant failure only 3 months later. These disappointing results prompted the investigators to conclude that GKRS did not show efficacy as an adjuvant treatment in the management of NGGCTs.

The study by Lekovic and colleagues[9] included 2 NGGCTs, one designated NGGCT and the other malignant teratoma. As with the other tumors in this series, the patients first underwent open biopsy and attempted GTR or debulking before institution of GKRS. The NGGCT received a peak dose of 30 Gy and the malignant teratoma a peak dose of 26 Gy. The NGGCT responded well to GKRS, with a complete response noted at 73 months; the teratoma showed a partial response at 15 months (see **Table 3**). GKRS in these cases was coupled with conventional EBRT, which the investigators believe may have contributed to the good response. Therefore the investigators conclude that GKRS may be useful as a constituent of multimodal treatment of these malignant lesions, but they caution against its use as a primary treatment.

The largest series of GKRS for NGGCTs before that of Mori and colleagues is reported by Hasegawa and colleagues[20] and features only 4 patients. Included in the study are a mixed GCT with malignant teratoma elements, a mixed GCT with teratomatous elements, an embryonal cell carcinoma, and an NGGCT (no specific disease is mentioned, diagnosis based on increased CSF markers). The mixed GCT with malignant teratoma underwent craniotomy with GKRS (Leksell Gamma Knife, Elekta, Tokyo) boost to residual tumor during craniospinal irradiation; this treatment was followed by chemotherapy. The maximum dose was 28 Gy and the marginal dose was 14 Gy. Partial tumor regression without dissemination was noted at 45 months. The second mixed GCT first received chemotherapy and then underwent craniotomy with partial resection. Whole ventricular irradiation followed with a boost to the pineal region. One year later, GKRS was given for tumor regrowth with a maximum dose of 24 Gy and a marginal dose of 12 Gy. The tumor appeared stable 4 months after GKRS. In the embryonal cell carcinoma case, fractionated radiotherapy was the initial treatment, which led to decreased tumor size. Two months later, there was evidence of tumor regrowth, leading to an additional dose of radiation along with chemotherapy. The tumor continued to grow, and GKRS with maximum and marginal doses of 32 and 16 Gy, respectively, was performed. The tumor progressed and the patient died 5 months later. In the final case, GKRS was the initial treatment based on an assumed diagnosis of germinoma with maximum and marginal doses of 28 and 14 Gy, respectively. Leptomeningeal dissemination was discovered 4 months later despite regression of the primary tumor. The patient underwent craniospinal irradiation and chemotherapy, with evidence of complete regression at 29 months after GKRS (see **Table 3**). Based on this narrow experience, the investigators conclude that aggressive therapy with conventional radiation and chemotherapy is the mainstay of initial treatment. GKRS is regarded as an adjuvant tool, especially as a boost to the local tumor and in prepubertal patients in whom GKRS may allow their total brain dose to be reduced.

Glial Tumors: Astrocytomas

Pineal region astrocytomas most often arise from the dorsal midbrain (tectal gliomas) and seem to behave in a benign fashion.[1] They are typically found in pediatric patients and managed by observation alone (if they cause obstructive hydrocephalus then this situation is addressed surgically). Radiotherapy is reserved for patients who are symptomatic or whose gliomas invade beyond the tectum. Chemotherapy can be used as an adjunct in these cases. Cases involving GKRS of pineal region gliomas are extremely rare in the literature.

A low-grade astrocytoma and an anaplastic astrocytoma are included in the series of Lekovic and colleagues.[9] The low-grade glioma received a maximum dose of 28 Gy and showed a complete response at 21 months. By contrast, the high-grade glioma received a peak dose of 24 Gy and showed widespread distant metastases at 5 months, leading to the patient's demise at 8 months. In both cases, GKRS was used as an adjuvant treatment in conjunction with conventional radiation. As the investigators state elsewhere, GKRS shows greater promise as an adjuvant therapy in lesions of low malignancy than it does in highly malignant tumors.

SUMMARY

- There are few studies that explore the efficacy of GKRS in treating pineal region tumors
- Those studies that exist have mainly used GKRS as an adjuvant therapy rather than as a primary treatment modality
- On the whole, GKRS is safe in the pineal region and effective for some tumors
- The most success with GKRS treatment of pineal region tumors has been with benign, or low-grade, lesions
- The most experience with GKRS is in the setting of PPTs, namely pineocytomas
- GKRS has shown safety and efficacy in LTC of pineocytomas, and has potential as a primary treatment modality

- The role of GKRS in pineoblastomas is poorly defined; although it may have some efficacy as an adjuvant treatment in LTC, it seems largely ineffective as a primary treatment and in preventing disseminated disease
- There are limited data on the benefits of GKRS in germinomas given the high success rate of conventional radiotherapy
- GKRS has shown efficacy as an adjuvant treatment in the management of germinomas, but it remains far from usurping the role of conventional EBRT
- NGGCTs are comprised of such diverse subtypes and are of such high malignant potential that GKRS seems to offer little benefit, even as an adjuvant therapy
- Pineal region astrocytomas are often low grade and so rare that GKRS has no current role in their management
- There is a significant need for larger studies and longer follow-up before GKRS becomes widely adopted in the treatment of pineal region tumors.

REFERENCES

1. Blakeley JO, Grossman SA. Management of pineal region tumors. Curr Treat Options Oncol 2006;7(6): 505–15.
2. Bruce JN, Stein BM. Surgical management of pineal region tumors. Acta Neurochir 1995;134:130–5.
3. Reyns N, Hayashia M, Chinot O, et al. The role of Gamma Knife radiosurgery in the treatment of pineal parenchymal tumours. Acta Neurochir 2006; 148:5–11.
4. Jooma R, Kendall BE. Diagnosis and management of pineal tumors. J Neurosurg 1983;58:654–65.
5. Bruce JN, Ogden AT. Surgical strategies for treating patients with pineal region tumors. J Neurooncol 2004;69:221–36.
6. Schild SE, Scheithauer BW, Schomberg PJ, et al. Pineal parenchymal tumors. Clinical, pathologic, and therapeutic aspects. Cancer 1993;72:870–80.
7. Mori Y, Kobayashi T, Hasegawa T, et al. Stereotactic radiosurgery for pineal and related tumors. Prog Neurol Surg 2009;23:106–18.
8. Kano H, Niranjan A, Kondziolka D, et al. Role of stereotactic radiosurgery in the management of pineal parenchymal tumors. Prog Neurol Surg 2009;23:44–58.
9. Lekovic GP, Gonzalez LF, Shetter AG, et al. Role of Gamma Knife surgery in the management of pineal region tumors. Neurosurg Focus 2007;23(6):E12.
10. Clark AJ, Ivan ME, Sughrue ME, et al. Tumor control after surgery and radiotherapy for pineocytoma. J Neurosurg 2010;113(2):319–24.

11. Deshmukh VR, Smith RA, Rekate HL, et al. Diagnosis and management of pineocytomas. Neurosurgery 2004;55(2):349–55.

12. Lutterbach J, Fauchon F, Schild SE, et al. Malignant pineal parenchymal tumors in adult patients: patterns of care and prognostic factors. Neurosurgery 2002; 51:44–56.

13. Fauchon F, Jouvet A, Paquis P, et al. Parenchymal pineal tumors: a clinicopathological study of 76 cases. Int J Radiat Oncol Biol Phys 2000;46:959–68.

14. Manera L, Regis J, Chinot O, et al. Pineal region tumors: the role of stereotactic radiosurgery. Stereotact Funct Neurosurg 1996;66(Suppl 1):164–73.

15. Konovalov AN, Pitskhelauri DI. Principles of treatment of the pineal region tumors. Surg Neurol 2003;59:250–68.

16. Matsutani M, Sano K, Takakura K, et al. Combined treatment with chemotherapy and radiation therapy for intracranial germ cell tumors. Childs Nerv Syst 1998;14:59–62.

17. Endo H, Kumabe T, Jokura H, et al. Stereotactic radiosurgery followed by whole ventricular irradiation for primary intracranial germinoma of the pineal region. Minim Invasive Neurosurg 2005;48(3):186–90.

18. Subach BR, Lunsford LD, Kondziolka D. Stereotactic radiosurgery in the treatment of pineal region tumors. Prog Neurol Surg 1998;14:175–94.

19. Kochi M, Itoyama Y, Shiraishi S, et al. Successful treatment of intracranial nongerminomatous malignant germ cell tumors by administering neoadjuvant chemotherapy and radiotherapy before excision of residual tumors. J Neurosurg 2003;99(1):106–14.

20. Hasegawa T, Kondziolka D, Hadjipanayis CG, et al. Stereotactic radiosurgery for CNS nongerminomatous germ cell tumors. Pediatric Neurosurgery 2003;38(6):329–33.

Index

Note: Page numbers of article titles are in **boldface** type.

Moving?

Make sure your subscription moves with you!

To notify us of your new address, find your **Clinics Account Number** (located on your mailing label above your name), and contact customer service at:

Email: journalscustomerservice-usa@elsevier.com

800-654-2452 (subscribers in the U.S. & Canada)
314-447-8871 (subscribers outside of the U.S. & Canada)

Fax number: 314-447-8029

Elsevier Health Sciences Division
Subscription Customer Service
3251 Riverport Lane
Maryland Heights, MO 63043

*To ensure uninterrupted delivery of your subscription, please notify us at least 4 weeks in advance of move.

Printed and bound by CPI Group (UK) Ltd, Croydon, CR0 4YY

12/10/2024

01773442-0001